DATE DUE	
DEC 1 5 1992		

OPPORTUNITIES IN
NUTRITION CAREERS

Carol C. Caldwell

Foreword by
Mel Zuckerman, President
Canyon Ranch Health
   and Fitness Resort

VGM Career Horizons
A Division of National Textbook Company
4255 West Touhy Avenue
Lincolnwood, Illinois 60646-1975 U.S.A.

Photo credits

Front cover: upper left, The Aerobics Center; upper right, Heartland Health and Fitness Retreat; lower left, lower right, Carol Caldwell, Canyon Ranch.

Back cover: upper left, Dairy Council of Arizona; upper right, Saint Mary's Hospital; lower left, University of Arizona Health Sciences center; lower right, Carol Caprione, National Restaurant Association.

ABOUT THE AUTHOR

Carol Caldwell is Director of Nutrition Services at Canyon Ranch Resort in Tucson, Arizona. She is responsible for managing professional staff with primary emphasis on development of services and materials for guest education and special programs. She is also involved in personnel decisions and quality assurance program development and evaluation.

She was previously nutrition consultant to El Dorado Hospital and Park West Health, P.C. to develop and implement patient nutritional assessment programs and group nutrition education. She also developed and implemented a nutrition program for the elderly and was employed as a clinical dietitian.

Ms. Caldwell received her B.S. and M.S. degrees at the University of Arizona, with major in nutritional sciences and minor in exercise physiology and rehabilitation. She is a member of the American Dietetic Association and of the Practice Group, Sports and Cardiovascular Nutritionists. Her major career interests include sports nutrition, and writing and editing in the areas of food and nutrition.

FOREWORD

Health care deliverers throughout the world are finally beginning to realize the essential role that diet and nutrition play in the prevention and treatment of illness and disease. The nutritional links to killing diseases such as cancer and heart disease, to eating disorders, obesity and chemical imbalances, to recent research on virtually every aspect of an individual's health and well–being, all make the role of the nutritional professional one of the most exciting "helping sciences" of the future.

For many years, nutrition as the science of food was never particularly compelling to people. After all, wasn't food simply the best–tasting combination of ingredients that one could ingest to ease hunger or to "reward" oneself?

But then, in the 1960s, Adele Davis profoundly stated: "We are what we eat."

Until that time few people had really thought about food as fuel for their bodies, or about food as having a cause–and–effect relationship to health and disease. Only in recent years have we become aware of the powerful role that nutrition plays in continuing good health and in the ultimate quality of life.

For the first time, we in America are becoming involved

in our own health. Individuals are saying, "I'm willing to take some responsibility for my health and the quality of my life." Then—through exercise, nutrition and stress management—these concerned individuals strive to maximize their own potential for good health.

One of the easiest ways to improve the way you feel is to learn about what you are putting into your body, and what effect it has on you. There are foods that keep you alert, foods that help you to sleep, foods that give you strength and endurance to compete and, most important, foods that keep your body fueled for the highest performance and best health possible.

Yet many in this country are not nutritionally aware. It is estimated that at least one–fifth of the American populace is on some kind of weight–loss diet (despite research that indicates dieting actually can aggravate weight problems)... that approximately 90 million Americans are overweight... and that more than 40 million Americans are considered clinically obese.

The long–term solution to these staggering problems is knowledge. That's why all these populations could benefit from professional nutrition services.

Research shows that knowledge about nutrition is the key to making healthy food choices. This means knowing the nutritional content of foods, how to balance the diet, how much to eat and when. Once we know what to do, behavior changes are far more likely to follow. It is this self–responsibility through improved health awareness that will revolutionize the future of public health.

Even though the preventive health care movement is still in its infancy, it is obvious that the health care deliverer of yesterday will not be the same deliverer of tomorrow.

The nutrition professional—the dietitian—will be at the forefront of this changing health care delivery system, working with doctors, physical therapists, exercise physiologists, clinical psychologists and others who specialize in the preventive approach to health.

How wonderfully fulfilling it is to work with nutrition professionals at the leading edge, providing the education and awareness that nourishes the inborn potential for health each of us possesses.

Mel Zuckerman, President
Canyon Ranch Health & Fitness Resort
Tucson, Arizona

INTRODUCTION

The primary focus of *Opportunities in Nutrition Careers* will be to present information of use to people who are considering the profession of dietetics. The nutritionist and the dietician are concerned with providing nutritional services to people. The dietitian is defined as a health-care professional, who holds credentials as a registered dietitian, who affects the nutritional care of individuals and groups in health and illness.

The work of the dietitian and the nutritionist includes the application of the science and art of human nutrition in helping people select and obtain food for the primary purpose of nourishing their bodies in health or disease throughout their life cycles.* ** The professional's participation may

---

*Baird, S. C., and Armstrong, R. V. L.: *Role Delineation for Entry Level Clinical Dietetics, 1980, Summary and Final Documents.* Chicago, The American Dietetic Association, 1981.
**Lanz, Sally, J.: *Introduction to the Profession of Dietetics.* Philadelphia, Lea & Febiger, 1983.

include nutritional assessment, client evaluation of nutrition intervention, nutrition education, consultation to food service and management, and application of the findings of current research.

THE SCOPE OF THE PROFESSION

To further understand the scope of the profession it is important to define the terms *nutrition* and *nutritional care.* These are terms which determine how the dietitian practices in various areas.

NUTRITION AS A SCIENCE AND AN ART

Nutrition is defined today as the science of food, the nutrients and other substances therein, their action, interaction, and balance in relation to health and disease, and the process by which humans ingest, digest, absorb, transport, utilize, and excrete food substances. In addition, nutrition must be concerned with social, economic, cultural, and psychological implications of food and eating.*

Nutritional care is the application of the science of nutrition. It is the art of helping people select and obtain food for the primary purpose of nourishing their bodies. It is essential both in health or disease throughout the life cycle.**

The goals of nutritional care are comprehensive. They include: improvement of the quality of life, prevention of disease, and clinical therapy during illness. To meet the goals of nutritional care, dietitians practice in many different settings—hospitals or other health–care facilities, schools and universities, business and industry, and community agencies. Dietetic practitioners can be involved in clinical practice, research, management of foodservice systems, food processing, communications, and teaching. Whether nutritional care is provided to improve the lives of individuals, manage a large–scale food operation, teach other health scientists and consumers or explain the nutritive content of food to children, the dietitian will be participating in many sophisticated and multifaceted roles.*

THE INCREASING ROLE OF NUTRITION

Because of the greatly increased interest in nutrition in recent years, the role of nutritionists and dietitians in our society is in a state of rapid growth and change. Only a few short years ago, the most basic principles of nutrition were largely unknown to the general public. Today, knowledge of the role of nutrition in human health is increasingly the subject of magazine and newspaper articles, books, television shows, and programs at public meetings. Movie stars, presidents, and other public personalities mention their health and fitness activities. Sports and athletic figures are quoted on how they maintain their diets and nutritional well–being.

Interest in nutrition is evidenced in food product commercials, and newspaper and magazine advertising. Demand for nutritional information on packaged food products has created a new policy, and product labels are increasingly specific about the nutritional worth of the products. Hospitals, doctors, and nurses are increasingly concerned about nutrition, and many have returned to medical schools for the latest information on nutrition and dietetics.

Nutrition courses in public schools, colleges, medical

---

*Pamphlet: *Dietitians: The Professionals in Nutritional Care.* Chicago, The American Dietetic Association.

schools, and other educational institutions are on the increase. The result of all this growth has been a flurry of new, widely varied, exciting courses available to the public and to the nutrition specialist.

THE PROFESSIONAL OUTLOOK

To the person who is presently considering a career as a nutrition professional, as a dietitian, a nutritionist, a teacher, or nutrition therapist, or any of a number of new specialties in this area, this is a time of exciting new opportunity. As the nutrition field grows in the next decade, more and more opportunities will open up. For some, this period of growth and change will actually mean pioneering in areas of human nutritional care that have not even been imagined today. Just as the health spa is no longer the privilege of just a few, good nutritional practices are no longer within the reach of only the privileged. The public is growing more and more aware of the opportunities for better health, and longer life, through the use of good nutritional practices—and the demand for professionals in this field will continue to expand along with this public awareness.

CONTENTS

Lecturer/writer/consultant. Professor/Nutritionist:
University of Arizona. Conclusion.

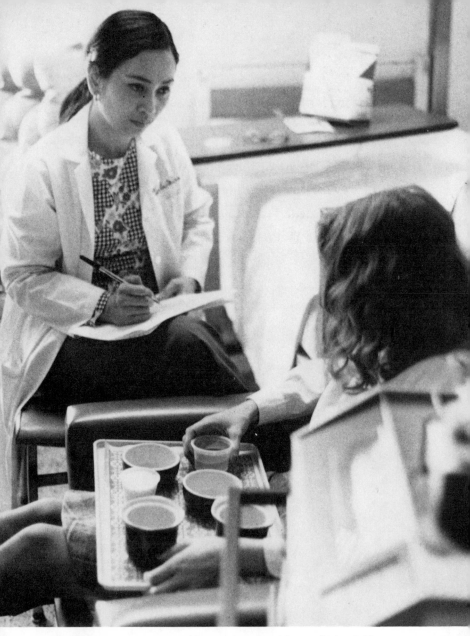

There are many opportunities open to a nutrition professional. The Registered Dietitian works in many areas of institutional health care. Photo: University of Chicago Medical Center.

CHAPTER 1

NUTRITION: A GROWING PROFESSION

It is an exciting time to be a nutrition professional. Never before have so many people been so visibly interested in nutrition.

This popular interest in the subject can be measured by the large number of best-seller diet books, as well as the fortunes being made by serving the public's desire for nutritional information and diet counseling, health books, and diet supplements.*

It is now apparent that optimal nutrition can be a strong factor in maintaining health and preventing disease. Physicians and other health professionals are recognizing the value of nutrition. The complexities of modern medicine demand high quality nutritional care services.

REASONS FOR CHANGE

Dramatic changes are occurring in the expanding nutrition profession. These changes arise from two new developments: (1) new computer applications in the nutrition field;

---

*The Dietitian—A Left-Over Role? *Journal of the American Dietetic Association* (81), December, 1982.

and (2) the general population's desire to know more about how nutrition affects them as individuals. The success of this field's expansion relies on the dietitian's ability to provide quality services to the public, at a time when the public is searching for accurate nutritional information and cost-effective health care.

Opportunities are available to the nutrition professional—the Registered Dietitian—to expand the practice environment. Dietitians may act as consultants to small community hospitals; long-term nursing care institutions; or special interest groups, such as sports trainers. In industry, they may be members of a product development or market research team, or they may be in the sales force. In public health, they may supervise nutritional programs for the elderly or for patients recently released from acute-care facilities. In the community, the dietitian can provide nutritional support or outpatient and in-home counseling services.*

BEFORE YOU ENTER THIS FIELD

Before entering this job market, it is critical to determine your individual interests. Dietitians in different types of settings have different types of experiences. Therefore, when you enter the job market you should consider what kind of experience you want before searching for a position.

The challenges the nutrition professional faces are exciting. It is a time when nutrition experts can create the world in which they work; but, it will take initiative, advanced knowledge, and the development of individual expertise. As

---

*Calvert, Susan, et. al. Clinical Dietetics: Fores Shaping Its Future. *J. Am. Diet. Assoc.* 80:350, 1982.

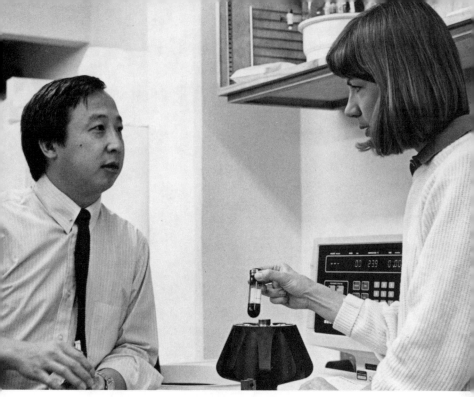

Much of the work in nutrition in the university setting is centered around research. Photo: University of Arizona, Department of Nutrition and Food Science.

a nutrition professional, you will find it a privilege to play a crucial role in this field; for nutrition is an essential component, not only of health and health care, but of life itself.*

---

*Young, Eleanor A.: Nutrition: An Integral Aspect of Medical Education. *J. Am. Diet. Assoc.* 82:490, 1983.

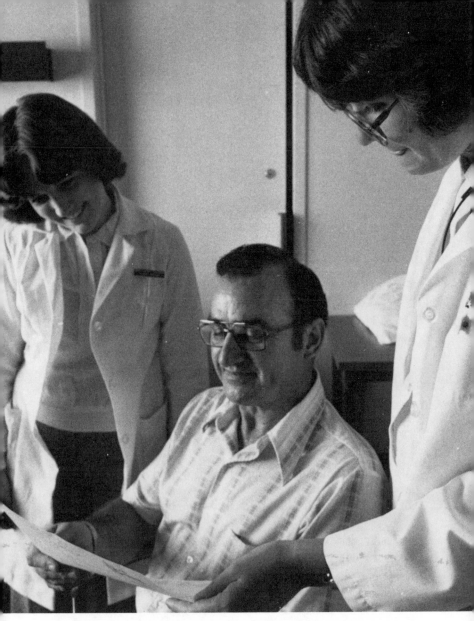

Dietitians often work directly with patients to counsel and plan nutrition programs. Most are members of the American Dietetic Association, and take part in continuing programs to maintain current skills and knowledge in the field. Photo: Iowa State University.

CHAPTER 2

THE AMERICAN DIETETIC ASSOCIATION: THE DIETITIAN'S HERITAGE

The profession of "Dietetics," as it is known today, began with the founding of the American Dietetic Association in 1917, under the direction of Lenna Frances Copper. She believed that there was a need for a conference to formulate a plan for dietetic communication. The first challenge faced by this new organization was how dietitians could best serve the nation's needs during World War I, both at home and overseas.*

ADMINISTRATION AND MANAGEMENT

Originally, administrative dietetics and food management were the specialties of the profession. The term "dietitian" was associated with those who worked in hospitals. Their objective was to provide quantity food production without loss of quality,** and to standardize institutional feeding.

---

*Horton, Loyal E., R. D.: The Boys in the Club. *J. Am. Diet. Assoc.* 81:17, 1982.
**Wilder, R. M.: The Hospital Nutrition Expert. *J. Am. Diet. Assoc.* 1:118, 1925.

DEVELOPMENT OF STANDARDS

During the second decade of the association, the dietitian was involved with support of government regulation and welfare agencies, food labeling, developing labor standards for commercial food service, and development of hospital food service plans. This dietetic movement was described as "one of the greatest existing forces in the promotion of health and the prevention of disease," but real advances would be achieved only when the results of nutritional research could be integrated into the practices of the population.*

By the 1940s, it had become clear that the profession needed to further develop standards in monitoring the quality of food, and to become involved in research to develop new food products. In addition, dietitians were involved in government efforts to develop nutritional standards for the school lunch programs.**

PUBLIC INFORMATION

During the 1950s the American Dietetic Association began a formal public relations program to strengthen the position of the dietitian, and to promote better understanding and recognition of the expertise of the dietitian. The dietitian was also urged to contribute to national health, research, and education. They were no longer only involved in food service and quality control but were expanding into all areas that nutrition could impact. These areas included government

---

*Turner, C. E.: Health Education as a World Movement. *J. Am. Diet. Assoc.* 12:457, 1936.
**Davis, B. D., Ph.D., R. D.: Quality & Standards—The Dietitian's Heritage. *J. Am. Diet. Assoc.* 75:409, 1979.

agencies, food industries, universities and schools, and public health education.

NEW METHODS, EDUCATION, AND RESEARCH

The next ten years was a time for the dietitian to seek new methods and adapt to changing conditions; a challenge which carried into each subsequent decade as the dietitian continued to search for new information, and improve the quality of life through nutrition.

In the 1970s, there was increasing participation in education and research. This decade saw the organization of dietetics into four major areas of practice which included *diet therapy, education, community nutrition,* and *administration.** Interest in legislation also became important as the profession recognized the need for licensing of the dietetic practioner.

EVALUATION AND CHANGE

Now, in the 1980s, it is a time of critical evaluation and change. The need for change has brought about the emergence of specialties among nutrition professionals. Because of this, 22 Dietetic Practice Groups have been established. Each group has its own standing rules, officers, newsletters, goals and budget.*

---

*Langholz, Edna P., R. D.: The President's Page: The Dietetic Practice Groups. *J. Am. Diet. Assoc.* 80:584, 1982.

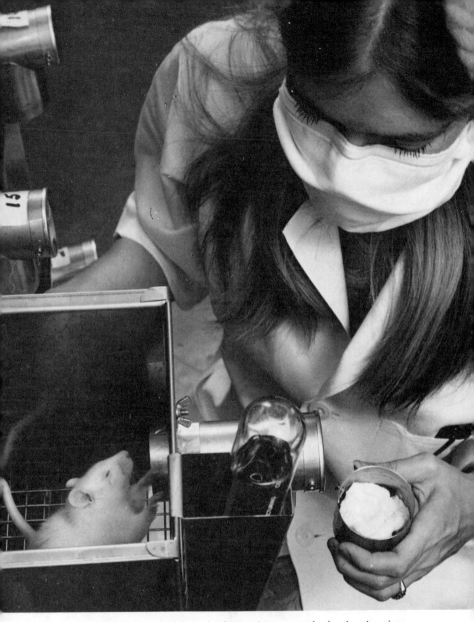

Above, a human nutrition scientist conducts research aimed at learning how the liver synthesizes fat from carbohydrates, information that may be related to coronary health in humans. Photo: United States Department of Agriculture.

CURRENT PRACTICE GROUPS

Public Health Nutritionists
Gerontological Nutrition
Dietetics in Developmental and Psychiatric Disorders
Community Nutrition Research
Research Dietitians
Renal Dietitians
Dietitians in Pediatric Practice
Diabetes Care and Education
Dietitians in Critical Care
Sports and Cardiovascular Nutritionists
Dietetics in Physical Medicine and Rehabilitation
Dietetics in General Clinical Practice
Consultant Dietitians in Health Care Facilities
Consulting Nutritionists–Private Practice
Dietitians in Business and Industry
ADA Members with Management Responsibilities in
    Health Care Delivery Systems
School Food Service
College and University Food Service
Dietetic Educators of Practitioners
Nutritionists in Nursing Education
Nutrition Education
Dietitians in Medical and Dental Education

These practice groups provide American Dietetic Association members with common interests and skills, and a chance to share ideas and expand their expertise.

The American Dietetic Association, along with the practice of dietetics, has expanded into all areas—new food development and preparation, weight management, the treatment and prevention of disease, research, nutrition for sports, and many others. Because of this dynamic growth, there are almost unlimited opportunities in the field of nutrition. The time for the nutrition professional is *now!*

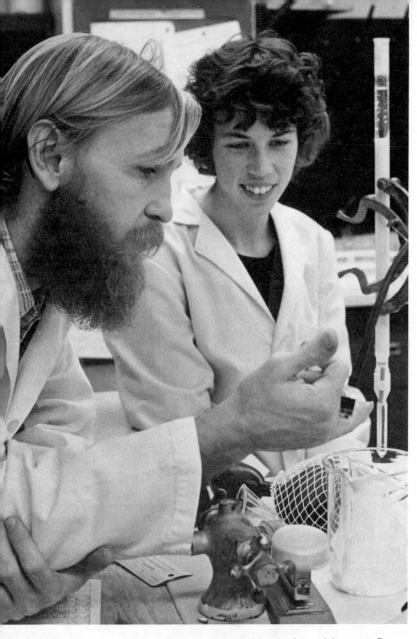
Above, a student and teacher in a nutritional sciences lab extract Beta-Carotene from spinach. Photo: New York State College of Human Ecology at Cornell University.

CHAPTER 3

DIETETIC EDUCATION

There are several education and experience routes which can be taken toward becoming a dietitian. The major education routes accredited or approved by the American Dietetic Association are *Plan IV Programs, Dietetic Internships, Coordinated Undergraduate Programs* (CUPs), and *Advanced Degree–with–qualifying–experience* programs.

The CUPs and Dietetic Internships are accredited by the American Dietetic Association, Commission on Accreditation (COA), in a process requiring site surveys. Programs in the other two pathways are approved by American Dietetic Association staff after a paper review; there is no formal accreditation of those programs.*

Each of these approved education programs will be discussed in detail in this chapter.

PLAN IV PROGRAM

This program consists of a formalized baccalaureate degree offered at an accredited college or university and is approved by the American Dietetic Association. (Note Appendix for a listing of the colleges and universities).

---

*Sullivan, Catherine Flood and Donald Smith. "Cost Effectiveness of Undergraduate Programs in Dietetics." *J. Am. Diet. Assoc.* 80:561, 1982.

11

Plan IV

MINIMUM ACADEMIC REQUIREMENTS
FOR ADA MEMBERSHIP

A Baccalaureate Degree Including Basic Requirements
Plus One Area of Specialization**

Area of Subject Matter	Basic Requirements	General
Physical & Biological Sciences	Chemistry, inorganic and organic Human physiology Microbiology	Biochemistry
Behavioral & Social Sciences	Sociology or psychology (principles) Economics	Cultural anthropology or sociology

[a]May be acquired prior to college entrance
[b]Recommended, not required
[c]If not completed in Basic Requirements
Adopted July 1, 1972
**Minimum Academic Requirements are expressed in terms of *basic competencies* rather than in specific credit hours. In *knowledge areas,* not in courses.

Areas of Specialization in Dietetics		
Management	*Clinical*	*Community*
	Biochemistry Biochemical analysis [b]Anatomy or [b]advanced physiology or [b]genetics	Biochemistry
Labor economics or relations	Cultural anthropology or sociology	Cultural anthropology or sociology [c]Psychology

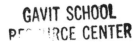

(Continued on next page.)

Area of Subject Matter	Basic Requirements	General
Professional Sciences	Food (composition, physical and chemical changes, quality, acceptability, and aesthetics) Prerequisite: organic chemistry Nutrition Prerequisites: human physiology & organic chemistry Management theory and principles	Food service systems management Nutrition in disease Prerequisite: biochemistry
Communication Sciences	Writing (creative or technical) [a]Mathematics to intermediate algebra) Learning theory or educational methods	[b]Data processing (computer logic) or [b]Data evaluation (statistics)

[a]May be acquired prior to college entrance
[b]Recommended, not required
[c]If not completed in Basic Requirements
Adopted July 1, 1972
**Minimum Academic Requirements are expressed in terms of *basic competencies* rather than in specific credit hours. In *knowledge areas*, not in courses.

Areas of Specialization in Dietetics		
Management	*Clinical*	*Community*
Food service systems management Principles of business organization (Management of personnel) Financial management	Additional nutrition course Prerequisite: biochemistry Nutrition in disease Prerequisite: biochemistry	Nutrition in disease Prerequisite: biochemistry Nutrition and community health Prerequisite: biochemistry Food service systems management (volume food service in the community)
Data processing (computer logic) or Data evaluation (statistics)	Data evaluation (statistics)	Data evaluation (statistics)

The Plan IV Program represents the current academic standards for the educational preparation of the professional dietitian. The faculty members of each college or university are responsible for evaluating the student's transcripts in terms of the institution's ADA–Approved Plan IV.*

The actual academic requirements for completion of Plan IV can be requested from the schools listed in Appendix.

DIETETIC INTERNSHIP

The Dietetic Internship is a formalized post–baccalaureate educational program. It is sponsored and conducted by various organizations outside of educational institutions and is accredited by ADA. Curriculums are designed to provide classroom and supervised clinical experiences to meet qualifications for dietetic practice. Students are required to enrole in an accredited internship following completion of the Plan IV Program to qualify for taking the written *Registration Examination.*

Entrance into Dietetic Internships are not guaranteed. The number of applicants is presently greater than the available positions. Therefore, it is important to be aware of the applicant selection processes.

The criteria for student selection used by most institutions include: a) academic record, which is the most heavily weighted; b) letters of recommendation; and c) student essays.

Academic Records. The grade point average (GPA) carries a relatively heavy weight. Educators view past academic success as a valid and reliable predictor of continued aca-

---

*Junkermier, Polly and Burness Wenberg. Implications of ADA Plan IV for Active Membership. *J. Am. Diet. Assoc.* 80:338, 1982.

demic success. Success in an internship program depends upon a firm academic base. Among the relevant subject areas, Science GPA's and English GPA's are considered good indicators of likelihood of success because of the strong emphasis on science, and written and oral communication skills in dietetics.*

Letters of Recommendation. These letters provide a means of learning about an individual's abilities in many areas. Most institutions usually request three letters, including character references from a professor in a major discipline, an academic advisor, a department chairperson, an instructor in a science course, or employers in professionally related jobs.*

Student Essays. These essays are used to gather information about an applicant's motivation, goals, and depth of interest in the profession. Typical essays include professional goals, reasons for choosing dietetics as a profession, reasons for choosing the institution's internship program and personal strengths and weaknesses.

An additional selection criterion includes work experience, to assure that the applicants have an understanding of the actual work performed and that they have a continuing interest in the profession. Volunteer work is as important as paid employment at this stage of the career.

Other selection variables include:

Conceptual Ability. Quality of written and oral expression, ability to master new information and skills, ability to understand complex new theory and to translate theory into practice are all important considerations.

---

*Brooks, Dorothy and Marie Dietrich. Student Selection in Dietetic Internship Programs. *J. Am. Diet. Assoc.* 80:355, 1982.

Overall Preparation. Relevance and quality of the applicant's previous educational experiences in school, in work, and in extracurricular activities; professionally related courses and electives taken as an undergraduate; refresher and/or advanced study done are also considered.

Self-direction. Ability to set goals, organize one's own activities, and work independently are essential skills.

Leadership Ability. Formal recognition of leadership through election to office and honors, and informal recognition by peers and others at school, work, and in extracurricular and community activities are indications of potential for success.

Ability to Perform Under Pressure. Flexibility, ability to set priorities, ability to set goals and organize work, physical stamina, and ability to remain reasonably calm under stress are evaluated. The overall load carried by student during college (academic, work, and extracurricular family or community responsibilities) is considered.

Interpersonal Skills. Realistic self–confidence, ability to sense the mood and concerns of others, appropriate use and interpretation of both verbal and nonverbal communications, ability to adapt to a variety of people and situations, and concern for the well–being of others are also important.*

COORDINATED UNDERGRADUATE PROGRAM (CUP)

The Coordinated Undergraduate Program (CUP) consists of four years of undergraduate study, with coordinated class-

---

*Bonberg, Barbara and Mary Carey. Dietetic Internship Selection Process. *J. Am. Diet. Assoc.* 80:459, 1982.

room and clinical experiences during the junior and senior years. The CUP program must follow specific guidelines for program assessment, development, implementation, and evaluation. Each must also meet prescribed standards for organization and administration, faculty and staff, facilities, and student services.

In contrast to the Plan IV Program, the clinical component for CUP is supervised by college or university faculty members and consists of 900 to 1000 clock hours. In the coordinated program, the need for an internship after graduation is eliminated. Thus, it takes five years to become professionally qualified in the Plan IV Program, but only four years in the CUP program.

ADVANCED DEGREE WITH QUALIFYING EXPERIENCE

A candidate must receive a Master's or a Doctoral Degree and complete a qualifying experience. This "experience" following completion of the Master's Degree consists of six months full–time or twelve months half–time work experience in the practice of dietetics. This experience should follow completion of current A.D.A. academic requirements. Two endorsements are required. One endorser must be involved in the academic or work experience for at least a six month, full–time continuous period, on the premise with the individual. At least one of the two endorsers must be a Registered Active ADA member for the past three years.

The qualifying experience following completion of a Doctoral Degree includes a six month experience in teaching, research, or practice in dietetics with endorsements the same as for the Master's Degree.

The education pathways discussed here may seem confusing. It is important as an interested nutrition student that you discuss your questions with a counselor knowledgeable in this area. As an example we will take a look at a typical educational and professional pathway of development.

Lee X. completed a Plan IV Academic Program at the University of Arizona. The course work completed was similar to that listed earlier in this chapter. Rather than immediately enter an Internship Program, Lee continued course work and received a Master's of Science in Nutritional Science with minor studies in Exercise Physiology and Rehabilitation. Then Lee developed a six-month, full-time work experience through St. Joseph's Hospital in Tucson. Lee's experience emphasized clinical dietetics with some work in community nutrition and food service administration. Lee's two endorsers were the Chief Clinical Dietitian at St. Joseph's Hospital and a major professor at the University of Arizona. After finishing the work experience, Lee sent a final report to the ADA which detailed the work experience. At that point, Lee was approved to take the written Registration Exam.

It is important to note that educational requirements in the field are under constant review and are subject to change. For the most up-to-date information at the time you are ready to make your plans, you should write to:

> The American Dietetic Association
> 430 North Michigan Avenue
> Chicago, Illinois 60611

You should ask for: *The Requirements For Membership in The American Dietetics Association* and/or *Eligibility for the Registration Examination For Dietitians.*

DIETETIC EDUCATION:
A CHANGING CLIMATE

As dietetic leaders project the future education of dietitians, it is realized that graduates of education programs must be prepared to perform the expected functions of the dietetic practitioner in a dramatically changing system. More then ever before, *education must be made relevant to practice.**

It is important for the students to develop an education program which will meet their individual needs and practice interests. More specifically, the student should be aware of the areas in education which should be strengthened based on current practice demand. These include a) a broader base, particularly in arts, humanities, and behavioral sciences; b) greater emphasis on management and business; c) greater emphasis on communications and networking; d) greater emphasis on new technology, especially the use of computers; and e) greater depth in scientific knowledge of nutrition.**

---

*Haschke, Marilyn and LTC Roy Maize. Dietetic Education: The Future and Policy Decision. *J. Am. Diet. Assoc.* 84:208, 1984.

**"A New Look at the Profession of Dietetics: Final Report of the 1984 Study Commission on Dietetics: Summary and Recommendations." *J. Am. Diet. Assoc.* 84:1052, 1984.

Zolber, Kathleen, "President's Page: Survival in the System." *J. Am. Diet. Assoc.* 81:594, 1982.

Turcotte, Judith Marie, Vaden, Allene G. and Donald P. Hoyt. Recommendations of the National Commission on Allied Health Education: Priorities for the Dietetic Profession. *J. Am. Diet. Assoc.* 83:533, 1983.

Fargen, Donna, Vaden, Allene G., and Richard E. Vaden. Hospital Dietitians in Mid-Career. *J. Am. Diet. Assoc.* 81, 1982.

Schwartz, N. E. and R. D. Gobert. Continuing Education in Nutrition and Dietetics: A working Model. *J. Am. Diet. Assoc.* 39:288, 1978.

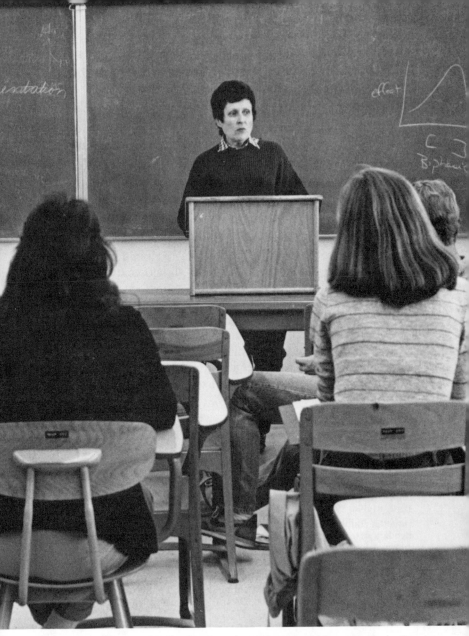

In addition to specific dietetic study, students should have courses in the behavioral sciences, management and business, and computers. Photo: University of Arizona, Department of Nutrition and Food Sciences.

It is apparent that education must meet the individual's needs and specialty interests. Open course work should focus on those areas which the students perceive as being important to their practice in the field. In addition, the student should seek volunteer work through hospitals, restaurants, resorts, out–patient facilities, nursing homes, etc. This will enable them to develop field experience to help determine realistic career objectives.

Dietitians of the future will not be able to serve as leaders unless the rigor and the credibility of their educational experiences are strengthened. The same is true for basic education programs, field experiences, advanced education in specialty areas, on–the–job training, graduate programs leading to advanced degrees, and continuing education.

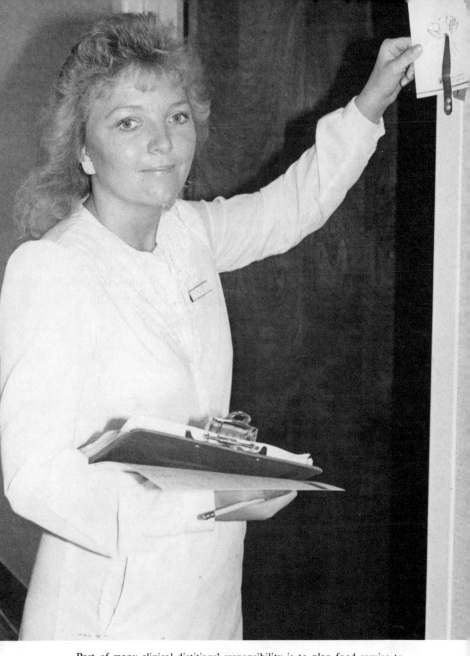

Part of many clinical dietitians' responsibility is to plan food service to hospital patients. Photo: Saint Mary's Hospital, Rochester, Minnesota.

CHAPTER 4

THE PRACTICE OF
CLINICAL DIETETICS

The clinical dietitian is defined as a health care professional credentialed as a Registered Dietitian, who affects the nutrition care of individuals and groups in health and illness. The clinical dietitian provides nutrition assessment; planning, implementation, and evaluation services; consultation to food service systems; and manages departmental and personnel functions for nutrition care services. The clinical dietitian also coordinates patient care as a member of the health care team, maintains and updates their individual skill and knowledge, and conducts applied research.*

Having thus defined the clinical dietitian, it is important to note also that these responsibilities are not necessarily performed by *every* clinical dietitian in *every* position. What will be discussed in this chapter deals with the entry–level clinical dietitian. Sub–specialities in clinical dietetics which require more specialized skills will be discussed later.

An entry–level position is defined as one that can be filled

---

*Baird, Shirley, Ed. D., R. D., et. al.: Role Delineation and Verification for Entry-Level Positions in Clinical Dietetics. Chicago, The American Dietetic Association, 1984.

by a practitioner with experience of three years or less. The following is included to provide information about the skills necessary to perform as an entry–level clinical dietitian. According to the American Dietetic Association, the responsibilities listed below are those the entry–level clinical dietitian will be able to perform.*

A. Plan and Organize

1. Use institutional and departmental standards to establish goals and priorities related to clinical nutrition, quality food, ethics, and education.
2. Participate in departmental program development using appropriate resources.
   a. Compare budget and accounting systems to institutional standards.
   b. Plan for computer utilization.
   c. Develop guidelines for work schedules.
   d. Develop policies and procedures.
   e. Review evaluation strategies.
   f. Assist with quality assurance planning.
3. Formulate an education plan.
   a. Plan for personnel training.
   b. Plan for nutritional and therapeutic needs of individuals and groups.
   c. Select principles and theories of education appropriate for the desired plan.

B. Gather and Evaluate Data

1. Assess nutritional needs of individuals and groups.
   a. Collect appropriate information for menu planning.
   b. Collect appropriate information on the patient through the use of the medical record, questionnaires, interview, community agencies, anthropo-

---

*Meredith, Susan, O.T.R., et. al.: Practitioner Competencies. *J. Am. Diet. Assoc.* 80:168, 1982.

metric measurements, intakes of food, nutrients, and fluids, and use of drugs.
c. Establish methods for client inquiry (i.e., client or family interviews to obtain information in relation to physical, emotional, environmental, economical, and cultural factors).

2. Perform accurate dietary calculations and evaluate appropriate application.
3. Demonstrate research techniques.
   a. Review current literature.
   b. Use resource materials effectively.
   c. Identify problems, issues, priorities.
   d. Select methodology for study.
   e. Implement methodology.
   f. Gather and evaluate data for use in improvement of program, system, or procedures.
4. Appraise potential of individual for employment and upward mobility based on application and interview.
5. Appraise employee for upward mobility based on performance evaluation.
6. Evaluate products in relation to availability, cost, quality and procurement.
7. Evaluate nutritional programs and services of private or tax-supported agencies.
8. Evaluate outcomes of patient education plan by assessing changes in food habits, teaching methods, and learner achievement.
9. Contribute and retrieve information from computer data storage.

Communicate and Report
1. Delegate responsibility to personnel in nutrition care and foodservice systems.
2. Communicate through verbal and nonverbal means in interviewing, counseling, and evaluating.

3. Communicate in writing clearly, concisely, and in understandable terminology.
4. Communicate professional expertise in classes, meetings, conferences and rounds.
5. Establish inter– and intradepartmental communication systems.
6. Conduct personnel training programs.
7. Develop, update, and interpret policies and procedures.
8. Monitor personnel utilization by evaluating workload of personnel and approving work schedules.

D. *Counsel and Supervise*–Apply principles of psychology, principles of management, and counseling skills in the supervision and motivation of personnel and clients.
   1. Identify problem areas with personnel/clients.
   2. Assist personnel and clients to identify alternative solutions and implement changes.
   3. Review progress with personnel and clients.

E. *Apply Scientific Principles—Foodservice Systems Management.*
   1. Establish standards for menu planning to coordinate with production and service.
      a. Approve regular and modified diet menus for nutrient adequacy, accuracy, and quality appropriate to individuals or groups.
      b. Evaluate menu cycle for changes.
   2. Monitor safety, security, and sanitation standards.
   3. Maintain budget controls.

F. *Apply Scientific Principles—Clinical Nutrition.*
   1. Apply principles of management and nutrition to provide nutritional care for clients.
      a. Direct and evaluate personnel in the provision of nutritional care.
      b. Modify expenditures to comply with budget.

    c. Assess nutritional status and devise an individualized nutrition care plan.

    d. Implement plan through supervision of patient care and provision of nutrition education and follow-up to client and family.

    e. Evaluate and revise plan as necessary.

2. Translate dietary modifications into menus.

    a. Evaluate client acceptance of food.

    b. Evaluate food quality, nutritional adequacy, and accuracy of dietary modification.

    c. Approve regular and modified diet menus for nutrient adequacy, accuracy and quality appropriate to individuals.

    d. Evaluate dietary products and supplements.

3. Monitor safety, security and sanitation standards.

4. Determine criteria for disease entities.

    a. Document nutritional care of client according to established criteria.

    b. Approve written documentation by dietetic technician.

    c. Conduct audits of medical records at designated intervals.

5. Utilize data for computer assisted systems.

    a. Menu planning and nutrient evaluation.

    b. Calculation of client nutrient intake and utilization.

    c. Client's medical data base.

    d. Criteria for audit.

6. Apply current nutrition research for improvement of program or system.

G. *Apply Scientific Principles in Community Nutrition*— principles of management and nutrition to provide nutritional care for clients in a program or agency.

1. Identify nutrition needs in the community.

2. Assess community resources.

H. Demonstrate Creativity
1. Apply creative and innovative methods and ideas.
   a. Solve problems.
   b. Merchandise products, services, nutrition, and the profession.
   c. Plan nutrition and foodservice programs.
   d. Develop educational methods and teaching aids.
2. Apply scientific principles using innovative methods in foodservice management, clinical nutrition, and community nutrition.
3. Continue to seek new ways of communicating with others.

I. Exhibit Professional Performance and Accountability.
1. Maintain registration as a professional dietitian.
2. Practice American Dietetic Association Code of Professional Practice and Guidelines for Professional Conduct.
3. Maintain a professional standard of practice.
4. Maintain current professional knowledge by reviewing the literature, maintaining updated resource files, participating in institutional and professional conferences and seminars, and writing technical reports, critical reviews, and articles.
5. Utilize problem solving methods.
6. Practice self–assessment and assessment of others by developing goals for improvement.
7. Integrate self into the professional role by applying interpersonal skills and assuming leadership roles in the profession.
8. Integrate own position and role into a program or system.
9. Promote departmental and program objectives.
10. Provide continuing education for staff and personal development based on needs.

11. Determine legal implications in the practice of dietetics and seek appropriate liability coverage.
12. Follow institutional policies for the protection of personnel and clients.
13. Seek information on current legislation affecting personnel, patient care, and the profession.
14. Comply with employer and institutional contracts, and government regulations.

These skills represent performance at an entry–level, showing depth of knowledge acquired; but, they do not indicate that all practitioners will utilize all skills.

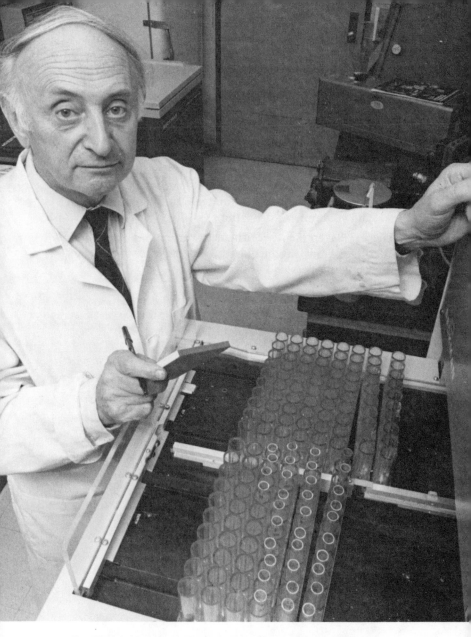

Dr. Hamish M. Munro, director of the Human Nutrition Research Center on Aging, does research in the area of protein metabolism. Photo: USDA.

CHAPTER 5

CLINICAL DIETETICS — SUB-SPECIALITIES

In this chapter we will discuss the various segments of clinical dietetics: research, pediatrics, critical care, physical medicine and rehabilitation, renal dietetics, diabetes and sports and cardiovascular nutrition. These sub–specialities broaden the scope of clinical dietetic practice and provide interested individuals an opportunity to become expert in a particular area.

It is interesting that the field of dietetics is becoming very specialized; as in the field of medicine where physicians often choose to specialize in one area. The clinical dietitian today is also expanding her or his skills in the development of a speciality, and many are becoming nutrition experts in highly developed areas.

RESEARCH DIETITIANS

Dietitians become specialized in this area through their work in clinical research centers and through public health projects. Most start out in general clinical practice and then go on to research, for which a Master of Science Degree is usually required. The research environment may be in a university, a hospital (in–patient and/or out–patient setting) or a public health setting.

Candidates interested in research work need to be careful, objective, and self–starters, with clinical experience. Additional training requires knowledge about grant writing to acquire money, scientific journal writing, and statistics.

Positive aspects of choosing a career in this area include the facts that one can work independently and with other high level professionals. Activity in research also demands the ability to combine and develop knowledge of many aspects of nutrition; e.g., biochemical, physiological, and psychological.

With substantial research training and experience, a Registered Dietitian can move from one area to another to do research, rather than staying in one specialization area.*

The future direction of research will probably focus on the effectiveness of nutritional intervention, as society focuses on the importance of preventive measures in terms of both cost and health effectiveness. Although the exact nature of the linkages between nutrition factors and health remains controversial, there appears to be a broad consensus that diet, nutrition, and eating habits are significantly related to health status.** These health issues will expand the opportunities available to the research dietitian.

---

*Meyering, Suzanne.: Discussion Paper #17-An Exploratory Study of Trends and Specialities in Clinical Dietetics. June, 1981.
**Talpin, Harriet.: Economics of Health Care. *J. Am. Diet. Assoc.* 76:218, 1980.

DIETITIANS IN PEDIATRIC PRACTICE

Dietitians enter pediatric practice because of the opportunity to work with children. Becoming specialized in pediatrics requires practice in a children's hospital or a hospital with a pediatric unit, or may require an advanced degree specializing in infant/child nutrition. Work settings vary, but usually the practitioner begins in a general hospital pediatric environment, and then moves on to do other pediatric work. These environments may include medical centers, hospitals, schools, day care centers, physician offices, and research centers.

Training for entry–level positions in pediatric practice include registration with 1–2 years experience in the sub–specialty area.

The demand for pediatric practitioners will be influenced by the birth rate, expanding child care programs, legislative trends, and technology. Another area which will impact pediatric practice will be the expanded focus on maternal nutrition to improve the outcome of pregnancy.* This area may extend the pediatric practitioner's involvement to include maternal and pre–natal care.

DIETITIANS IN CRITICAL CARE

Dietitians in critical care have a strong therapeutic background, typically working in a university or teaching hospital providing care to the critically ill patient. Most have obtained a Master's Degree or advanced training beyond the clinical internship. Positive features of this specialty include increased contact with medical staff, opportunities for research, teaching, and publishing.

---

*Hughes, Mary.: Healthy Mothers, Healthy Babies. *J. Am. Diet. Assoc.* 80:215, 1982.

Critical care dietitians work with parenteral and enteral nutrition, nutrition assessments, and drug–nutrient interactions. They also work closely with patients to improve nutritional status.

Sub–specialities in this area are increasing due to the importance of nutrition in critical illness and the specifics of nutrition therapy. These sub–specialities include nutrition support services, oncology (the scientific study and treatment of tumors), hematology (the science dealing with the formation, composition, functions and diseases of the blood; i.e., anemia), neonatology (the scientific study and treatment of newborns), and advanced burn centers.*

These specialities involve high pressure work environments and long hours which demand leadership, assertiveness and career commitment from the dietetic professional.

RENAL DIETITIANS

Renal dietetics deals with the nutrition therapy of those individuals with kidney problems. Training for this specialty area requires clinical experience with advanced training, usually on a renal unit in a hospital or dialysis center.

Registered Dietitians interested in practicing in this area require special traits to handle intense, long–term patient care, including their psychological and sociological needs. They must be dedicated and have an interest in maintaining current educational status. Rapid change in knowledge in this area requires constant, continuing education.

Major work activities of renal dietitians include patient and family education, development of teaching materials,

---

*Roper, Nancy. *New American Medical Dictionary*. Churchill Livingstone, New York. 1978.

participation in medical rounds, interpretation of laboratory tests, and nutrition education of allied professionals. These responsibilities require knowledge about food composition, drug–nutrient interaction, and fluid electrolyte management in the body.

DIABETES CARE AND EDUCATION

Dietitians specializing in this area usually work in out–patient facilities or in–patient programs provided by hospitals. The required education includes a Bachelor of Science Degree with registration status. Additional course work or a Master's Degree is not required, but is helpful due to the complexity of the disease.

Diabetes care requires long–term treatment and patient education. This provides the dietitian with an opportunity to develop individualized long–term care, and follow the patient and family for an extended time. The dietitian will develop nutrition care plans, and educate the client regarding nutrition, psychosocial problems, and exercise. Diabetes care also enables the dietitian to work as a team member.

Opportunities in this area will probably expand due to the increased incidence and increasing knowledge of the disease. Also, technology will continue to shape this area of practice, as research and computers continue to affect methods of treatment.

SPORTS AND CARDIOVASCULAR DIETITIANS

Dietitians in this area usually begin with a clinical background as a Registered Dietitian, and then obtain a Master of Science Degree in Nutrition and Exercise Physiology.

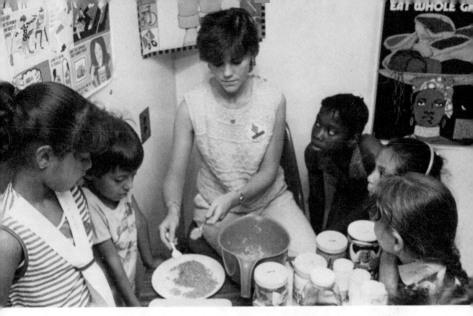

New York's Floating Hospital provides nutrition education programs and activities to all ages, in a unique setting on shipboard. Photos: The Floating Hospital, New York, New York.

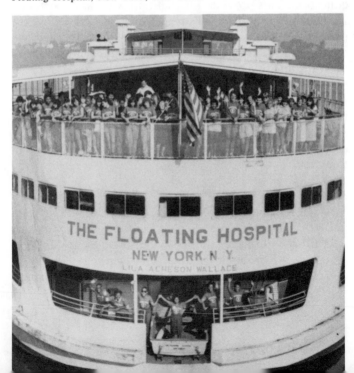

YMCA's, schools, universities, and businesses all provide a variety of opportunities to practice. This area will see the greatest expansion in the future due to the increased awareness of business, industry, and the general public about the importance of nutrition and exercise.

Candidates are drawn to this area because of a personal interest in sports and because clients are actively seeking nutrition information. The challenge in this area of practice is that dietitians must develop their own standards of practice, and create the structure of their work environment, because there are few guidelines yet developed in this new field.

Work activities include individual diet/nutrition counseling, development of education materials and audio–visual aides, computer nutrient analysis, writing, and research.

As more is learned about the combined importance of nutrition and exercise, the demand for dietitians in this area will increase, and their work environments will expand to include hospitals, the community, and specialty work in professional and amateur athletics.

CONCLUSION

Many of these clinical sub–specialities require advanced training after registration, which includes a Master of Science or Ph.D. Degree, and significant work experience within the specialty area. This trend will continue as research and technology expand the "science" of dietetics and nutrition. Also, dietitians will do more independent research, develop policies and procedures, and consult and teach individuals and groups.

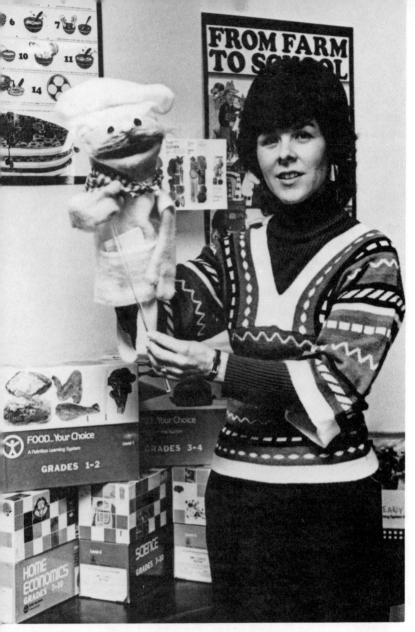

The community receives nutrition education from many sources today. These may include government, school, industrial, and commercial programs. Photo: Dairy Council of Arizona.

CHAPTER 6

COMMUNITY DIETETICS

The dietitian in a community setting plays an important role as a member of the health care team. The community dietitian becomes the translator of the science of nutrition into the skill of furnishing optimal nourishment to people. As the nutrition translator, the dietitian is educated in providing nutrition information, in interpreting nutrition facts accurately, and in using terminology that the public can understand and apply.*

The community dietitian is defined as a dietetic professional in a community who provides the nutrition services to individuals and groups. As a member of a team providing health care and nutrition services, the community dietitian performs nutritional assessment; and organizes, coordinates, and evaluates selected components of nutrition services for an organization or group.**

---

*Position Paper on recommended Salaries and Employment Practies for Members of The American Dietetic Association, *J. Am. Diet. Assoc.* 78:61, 1981.

**Baird, Shirley C. and Sylvester, J.: Role Delineation and Verification for Entry-Level Positions in Community Dietetics. Chicago, The American Dietetic Association. 1983.

Areas of sub–specialty in community nutrition include home health care, health maintenance organizations, private practice and business and industry.

HOME HEALTH CARE

The community dietitian will often provide nutrition services to clients in their homes. Usually a referral is made from a hospital health team to the dietitian. The dietitian reviews the patient's medical record, takes dietary history, assesses the patient's nutritional status, records food likes and dislikes, and develops a nutritional care plan based on pertinent information contributing to nutritional care.* The nutrition care plan will then help determine what services the dietitian will provide. These services may include: assessment of dietary intake by computer nutrient analysis; consultation with physicians prescribing diets; client and family counseling; follow–up conferences and in–service education with nurses, therapists, and home health aides; and the recording, reporting, and monitoring of progress and results of nutritional care.**

Once developed, the plan is then discussed with the client or home sponsor for the client. Issues which may arise in relation to home care may include: weight gain from overeating, lack of exercise, and complications in medical conditions. It is important to maintain contact with other health

---

*Oller, Juli A.: The Dietitian in Community Home Programs. *J. Am. Diet. Assoc.* 76:267, 1980.
**Hamilton, Louise W.: The President's Page. *J. Am. Diet. Assoc.* 75:460, 1979.

team members, and the community dietitian may need to expand the care plan, as the case proceeds.

The dietitian, by maintaining contact with the other health care providers can identify specific problems and refer them to the team member responsible for that area of specialization. In addition, "mini" home nutrition courses can be provided which focus on different areas of nutrition. The dietitian may provide sample menus for normal and modified diets, depending on the client's life style and medical therapy. The dietitian, therefore, needs to be aware of food costs, who purchases the food, cultural food preferences, and food preparation facilities. In this way, home visits provide an opportunity for the dietitian to identify socio–economic problems and then to determine instructional techniques to use in gaining acceptance and adherence to the diet and nutrition care plan.

Although not all clients need nutrition services provided in the home, many clients do need the assistance of a dietitian, including:

1. Those whose conditions have just been diagnosed and for whom a therapeutic diet is prescribed as part of their treatment.
2. Those who must make major diet changes.
3. Those who have been assessed as requiring assistance (e.g., a malnourished person on a fixed income who needs instruction and diet modification to increase protein and caloric intake).
4. Those whose disease symptoms recur due to poor comprehension of their diet.
5. Those who have been referred by a hospital/nursing home dietitian upon discharge from these facilities.
6. Those whose physician has requested a nutrition consultation, but who have no access to facilities due to

inadequate transportation or inability to travel long distances.*

The career benefits of providing home health care nutrition services are many. Home health care provides the ability to develop a long-term care plan for the client and to provide continued follow-up. The dietitian performs independently and also as a team member, and is responsible for the development of educational materials for client use.

The future for a community dietitian providing home health care is promising. Based on a survey done by The American Dietetic Association, only 300,000 to 500,000 people in the United States receive home health care services, although 1.7 to 2.7 million people are in need of these services. In addition, the dietitian, by providing home health services, may reduce total cost of providing health care. Examples of potential cost savings are:

1. Reducing need for rehospitalization because of malnutrition, uncontrolled diabetes, and so forth.
2. Preventing fractures due to disorientation or weakness related to malnutrition.
3. Delaying kidney dialysis treatment.
4. Preventing food poisoning from improper food sanitation at home.
5. Permitting earlier discharge of patients with parenteral or enteral feedings.
6. Assisting the patient to understand and use new technologies, thus preventing or delaying reinstitutionalization.
7. Hastening healing of postoperative patients.
8. Using a trained professional who is more efficient and

*Comments Related to a Study of Methods for Improving Coverage of Registered Dietitian's Services Provided by Home Health Agencies. *J. Am. Diet. Assoc.* 80:464, 1982.

accurate in the adjustment and readjustment of individualized diets.

Educational requirements include entry–level status and 2–3 years experience in a clinical setting. An advanced degree (M.S.) is preferred.

HEALTH MAINTENANCE ORGANIZATIONS

Health Maintenance Organizations (HMOs) are comprehensive medical facilities where, through an employer, families and/or individuals prepay for health care.* HMOs were developed to restructure health care delivery systems to provide equitable, high quality care for all; provide optimal utilization of health personnel; control costs; and satisfy consumers.** They are designed to bring together health services which individuals and families are most likely to need, for a fixed premium paid in advance by subscribers. An HMO is dedicated to providing: a) comprehensive care, defined as a full range of health services with emphasis on prevention; b) care continuity, coordinated on a family basis, throughout each member's life cycle and health–sickness cycle; and c) care that is organized and carried out to give maximum health service for the consumer dollars.***

---

*Rogasner, Marjorie.: Development of Health Maintenance Organizations and Use of Dietitians in HMOs—Discussion Paper #14. *The Dietetic Manpower Demand Study,* The American Dietetic Association. May, 1981.

**Health Maintenance Organizations, Concept and Strategy. *Hospitals.* 45:53, Mary 16, 1971.

***The American Dietetic Association Position Paper on Nutrition Services in Health Maintenance Organizations. *J. Am. Diet. Assoc.* 60:317, 1972.

The basic principle by which HMO operations will be successful lies in keeping people well, in order to avoid the more complex and costly services needed to treat illness and return them to health. In this way, the HMO provides a medical setting outside of the hospital where a dietitian can develop a varied practice and become more involved with each client by providing follow–up care.

Dietitians in this area are diet counselors, health educators and program evaluators. The dietitian deals both with individuals and families, as well as the health care team to provide total health services. In the role of diet counselor, the dietitian provides diet therapy to diabetics, cardiovascular patients, hypertensives and diet therapy during and following pregnancy. As the health educator, the dietitian teaches self–care, using nutrition as a framework to build positive behavior patterns. The dietitian may also be involved in specialty clinics to deal with obesity, alcoholism, smoking cessation and weight reduction. As a program evaluator, the dietitian has the opportunity work with HMO administrators to initiate new and evaluate on–going programs.

Nutrition services in an HMO, as suggested by the American Dietetic Association may be as follows:

PHASE OF HMO OPERATION	NUTRITIONAL CARE GOAL	NUTRITIONAL CARE ACTIVITIES*
Health appraisal and referral	To identify potential problems and plan for continuing surveillance or appropriate care	Assessment of food practices and nutritional status. Referral for corroboration. Data input into patient information systems.
Environmental protection and disease prevention; health maintenance	To prepare patients and their families to assume responsibility for	Individual counseling. Group teaching. Development and/or evaluation of nutri-methods and materials. Training and

---

*The American Dietetic Association Position Paper on Nutrition Services in Health Maintenance Organizations. *J. Am. Diet. Assoc.*

	their own care and to manage early symptoms to prevent complications	continuing education for medical, dental, and other professional staff; technical consultation. Training and continuing education for dietectic supportive personnel. Referral to, and liaison with, food assistance and other nutrition-related community programs. Leadership in seeking solutions to community-wide nutrition problems. Consultation to group care facilities.
Acute and intensive care	To develop and implement immediate and long–range individualized nutritional care plans for in– or out–patients	Most of the activities described above. On–going participation in health team planning, direct nutritional assessment and counseling, and evluation. Planning and/or supervision of appropriate group food service. Health team staff conferences. Initial and follow-up counseling in regard to normal and therapeutic nutritional needs. Input into clinical records.
Restoration and extended care	To assist patients and their families with long-term health problems to attain and maintain adequate diets	Most of the activities described above. Assistance in adjusting home environment to maximize independent functioning in activities in and outside the home. Liaison with non-contact services or programs helpful in carrying out the nutritional care plan.

Nutritional care activities clearly will overlap and seldom will be restricted to a single phase of operation.

The education required of the dietitian is at minimum a baccalaureate degree and is registered; a Master's Degree is suggested. The training in research and analysis that a Master's Degree level person has, provides the dietitian with more credibility and an increased opportunity for input into planning programs at the HMO.

Also helpful is knowledge of, and experience in, community organization and community health services and resources in order to provide counseling and direction in planning and implementing nutritional care. The dietitian should also be capable of training and supervising dietetic personnel and coordinating nutrition programs with other health care services.

Job satisfaction in this area is high because dietitians are occupying positions where they are gaining respect and credibility and public confidence. However, the R.D. must become more visable to other health care personnel, be able to "sell nutrition" and explain why it is important that they become part of the medical/health care team.

The future impact of HMOs on the dietetic profession is promising. According to the market research firm of Frost and Sullivan, Inc., the HMO "will emerge ... as a viable growing component in the U.S. health care system". It projects membership to increase to 24 million, about 13 percent of the population by 1990. This growth will provide dietitians with increased opportunity to practice in this area and establish their credibility.

DIETITIANS IN PRIVATE PRACTICE

A consultant dietitian is defined by the American Dietetic Association as a practitioner who "affects the management of human effort and facilitating resources by advice or service in nutritional care". The consultant is a dietitian in private practice whose services are utilized by nursing homes, other institutions, individuals, and groups.*

According to the ADA, the following are suggested roles the consulting dietitian performs:

A. Services provided to businesses or groups
   1. Evaluates and monitors food service systems, making recommendations to provide nutritionally adequate food.
   2. Develops budget proposals and recommends procedures for cost controls.
   3. Plans, organizes, and conducts orientation and inservice educational programs for food service personnel.
   4. Plans layout design and determines equipment requirements for food service facilities.
   5. Recommends and monitors standards for sanitation, safety, and security in food service.
   6. Develops menu patterns.
   7. Develops, maintains, and uses pertinent record systems related to the needs of the organization and the consultant dietitian.
   8. Provides guidance and evaluation of the job performance of dietetic personnel.
   9. Maintains effective verbal and written communications and public relations, inter- and intradepartmentally.

B. Services provided to individuals–
   1. Assesses, develops, implements, and evaluates nutritional care plans and provides for follow–up, including written reports.

---

*Lang, Sally J.: Introduction to the Profession of Dietetics. Philadelphia, Lea and Febiger, 1983.

2. Consults and counsels with clients regarding selection and procurement of food to meet optimal nutrition.
3. Develops menu patterns.
4. Develops, uses, and evaluates educational materials related to services provided.
5. Consults with the health care team concerning the nutritional care of clients.
6. Interprets, evaluates, and utilizes current research relating to nutritional care.

Education and experience necessary to practice as a consultant dietitian include:
1. Registration (R.D.)
2. One to four years of clinical or community nutrition experience.
3. A master's degree in business and/or nutritional sciences is not required but suggested.*

The dietitian in private practice will carry over into career areas already discussed and those to follow. These areas provide population groups where consultant dietitians can market their services.

As an example, a consultant might become involved in the employee health service of a corporation. For economic reasons, corporations are focusing on preventive health care and education to decrease health care costs and increase worker productivity. By changing the employee's "health profile", a corporation can save money by cutting sick time, decreasing the use of medical care, and avoiding early retirement due to disablement.**

Other areas for development of a private practice include:

---

*The New York Academy of Medicine and The New York Dietetic Association.: Physicians Give Consulting Dietitians the Nod. *J. Am. Diet. Assoc.* 75:531, 1978.

**Clutterbuck, D.: Executive Fitness Aids Corporate Health. *Internal Management.* 35:19, 1980; Popkin, B. M., Kaufman, M., and Hallahan, I. D.: The Benefits and Costs of Ambulatory Nutritional Care and Costs and Benefits of Nutritional Care, Phase 1. Chicago, American Dietetic Association, 1979.

— A physician's office or physician's group
— Nursing homes/Hospices
— Psychologist's groups
— Dental offices
— Weight–loss clinics
— Sports facilities

To facilitate practice in these areas as well as others, the dietitian must determine; a) the needs and interests of employees and clients regarding nutrition, b) design of counseling sessions, c) advertisement avenues which will most effectively sell the service, d) method of client referral, e) additional resources available for client education, f) other competition, and g) fees, considering costs required to provide a "good" service and fringe benefits.*

Actual services provided may include:

1. Weight reduction, weight maintenance, or weight gain nutrition counseling.
2. Nutrition education.
3. Obesity, diabetes, cardiovascular disease treatment.
4. Bulemia/anorexia counseling.
5. Premenstrual syndrome therapy.
6. Smoking cessation counseling and therapy.
7. Substance abuse nutrition therapy.
8. Publishing for newspapers and magazines.

The positive aspects of a career as a consultant include the ability to sell oneself, developing an assertive, business profile; respect as a health professional from the medical community and also the public; and the challenge to succeed on your own. Some drawbacks may be the financial risk, and having to rely on physician referral for patients. Also, payment for service is often not insurance–reimbersible, and the general

---

*Seidel, Miriam C., R.D.: The Consulting Nutritionist in an Employee Health Office. *J. Am. Diet. Assoc.* 82:405, 1983.

public lacks the knowledge to understand exactly what the dietitian can provide.

Although there are obstacles as a consultant, the highly self-motivated dietitian can develop a successful and rewarding independent practice. This community sub–specialty will continue to expand as the general public becomes more aware of dietetic services and the importance of nutrition in maintaining health.

DIETITIANS IN BUSINESS AND INDUSTRY

This may be considered the area with the most rapid growth. In the past, dietitians in business and industry typically worked for food companies developing new food products. Now, as "wellness" becomes a prominent focus in the private sector, opportunities for the dietitian seem limitless.

Industry recruiters, as well as executives in food service management companies, report a continual need for dietitians in this area, especially those with management skills.* Many businesses hire dietitians for their technical expertise, providing the company with a competitive edge in marketing their products and services.

To take advantage of the opportunities available, dietitians need to expand their skills to include: a) management training, especially finance and marketing; b) oral, written and media communication skills; and c) the ability to "sell" oneself to promote ideas, new projects and to improve the image of the profession.

---

*Dowling, Rebecca.: Technical Report #4—Demand for Dietitians in Business and Industry. The Dietetic Manpower Demand Study: The American Dietetic Association, February 1981.

Recruiters and employers in this area are looking for the dietitian profile which projects:

—self–confidence in professional knowledge and ability to learn new information.
—an enthusiastic attitude about job and about working.
—achievement–orientation.
—assertive behavior in promotion of self, ideas, and products or services of employing corporation.
—willingness to travel or relocate.
—good communication skills.
—willingness to work long hours to accomplish a job.
—ability to utilize criticism for personal and professional growth.
—interest in upgrading and developing skills for advancement through a variety of continuing education programs.

The education required for an entry–level position in business and industry includes a B.S. from an approved dietetic program, registration, and management course work. Management experience is valuable but *not* necessary in all cases. Also, coursework in accounting and personnel management is suggested. For the dietitian wanting to move into a middle or top management position, a Master's in Business Administration (MBA) is becoming necessary.

Specific skills and knowledge required when entering business and industry include finance, writing and communication skills, marketing, public speaking, personnel management, budgeting and accounting, economics, food sciences, long–range planning and time management, and cost containment.

Types of positions available to the dietitian interested in practicing in business and industry include:

—Advertising, public relations and marketing
—Anthropology research
—Architects, or consultants to materials managers
—Chemical laboratory representatives
—Consumer affairs
—Cooking school instruction
—Equipment companies—service and sales
—Fitness and wellness centers, resorts and spas
—Food brokers and distributors
—Hospital administration and management
—Lawyer involved with nutrition regulations, codes, and labor
—Nursing
—Personnel directors
—Pharmaceutical companies—sales, product development, marketing
—Product development—food and equipment
—Production manager
—Restaurant management
—Retail stores—food demonstration and cookware sales
—Social/nutrition programs—development, evaluation, and management

Specific sub-specialty areas in this field are emphasized below.

JOBS WITH FOOD PRODUCT COMPANIES

Food product companies hire dietitians to serve as advisery staff to corporate management on nutrition related issues in product development, labeling, advertising, legislation, public relations, marketing and consumer education. Skills necessary beyond technical expertise include skills in human relations, the desire to excel, flexibility, and good oral and written communications skills.

JOBS WITH SALES COMPANIES

Sales companies utilize dietitians for their technical expertise regarding diet modification and food production and distribution. Dietitians have excellent opportunities as sales representatives because of their familiarity with the food and medicine industry. They have knowledge about medical therapy, know the language; and, therefore, can use a "soft-sell" approach. Additional skills required beyond technical expertise include skills in marketing, accounting, financial analysis, labor relations, and economics.

JOBS WITH FITNESS AND WELLNESS CENTERS

Fitness and wellness centers, resorts and spas utilize dietitians for their menu planning and diet modification skills, as well as client nutrition education and writing for popular press, newsletters, and educational material development. This area requires additional knowledge in marketing, finance, public relations, writing, accounting and a well-rounded nutrition background which focuses on health maintenance.

JOBS WITH BUSINESS AND INDUSTRY

Business and industry is presently the least defined career area. This can be a positive condition, however, because

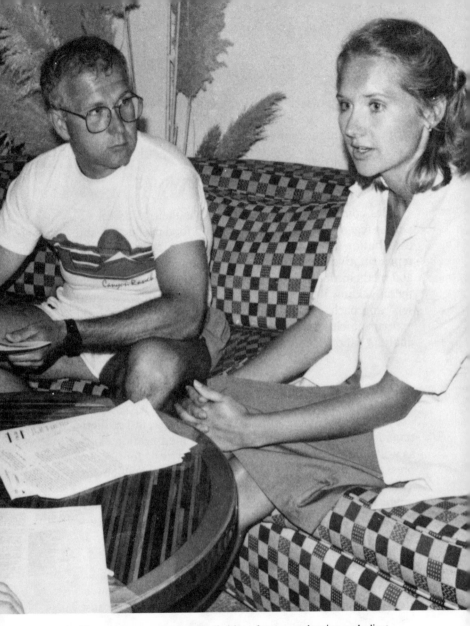

Fitness centers and spas use dietitians for menu planning and client services such as discussing diet modification and nutritional education. Here, the author (at right) meets with clients. Photo: Canyon Ranch Resort.

dietitians are able to develop their own policies and procedures and their practice environment. Corporate executives in foods companies, food service, and related industries are recognizing the valuable contributions of dietitians; some are viewing dietitians as candidates for middle- and upper-level management positions. In addition, the demand for qualified practitioners currently exceeds the supply. To become qualified, the dietitian must expand the breadth of dietetic training into business areas to aid in the development of the ability to market one's expertise and succeed in the business environment.

CONCLUSION

Community dietitians will increasingly be challenged to demonstrate specialized competencies and meet the total needs of the community. However, due to the unique role the dietitian may play as a health team member, opportunities will continue to expand—the future in community dietetics is bright.

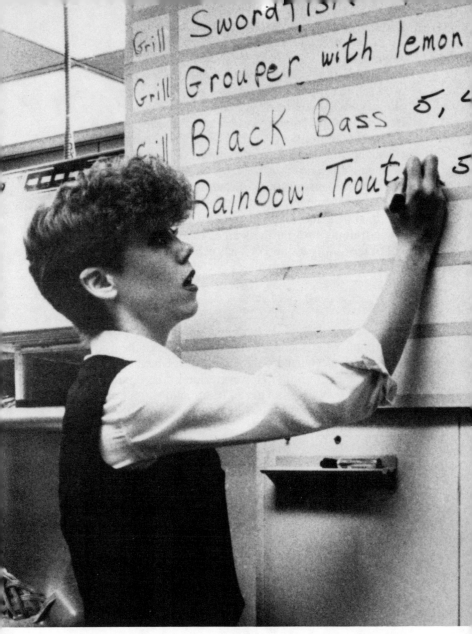

An administrative dietitian can be responsible for meeting all the objectives of a food service system from menu planning to service. Photo: National Restaurant Association.

CHAPTER 7

FOODSERVICE SYSTEMS MANAGEMENT: THE ADMINISTRATIVE DIETITIAN

Many nutrition professionals are entering the field of Foodservice Systems Management. Here there is a need for the administrative dietitian, a management specialist. This area of dietetic practice includes many administrative and management responsibilities. Also, technologic, social, and economic developments in food service are making well-qualified foodservice administrators more necessary than at any previous time.* Although this area may not sound dynamic, it has opportunities available for management growth, long–term job security and benefits, and the ability to develop experience that can be applied in other fields.

Management is the major function of the administrative dietitian; specifically foodservice systems management. This area of management is defined as the process of accomplishing food service system objectives. These include menu planning, food procurement, production, distribution, and service. Through integration of resources within the total food

---

*Lanz, Sally J. Introduction to the Profession of Dietetics. Philadelphia, Lea and Febiger, 1983.

system and by working with and through individuals and groups, these objectives are met.*

The roles performed by the entry–level dietitian in food-service systems management are delineated below. These represent a combination of actual roles, which currently exist, and those which ought to exist. These roles are abstracted from the *Role Delineation Study for Foodservice Systems Management* published by the American Dietetic Association.

The foodservice systems management professional:

1. Focuses foodservice operations on nutrition goals of a target market.
2. Advances practitioner competence through self–improvement programs.
3. Promotes positive working relationships with others whose work has an impact on foodservice systems.
4. Utilizes current foodservice systems and nutrition information in management and research.
5. Manages foodservice sub–systems, including food procurement, production, distribution, and service.
6. Manages foodservice system resources, including human, material, physical, and operational assets.
7. Manages Quality Assurance Programs in area of responsibility.
8. Advocates action which advances foodservice systems management and improves nutrition status of consumers.**

---

*Baird, Shirley C., and Sylvester, Joan.: Role Delineation and Verification for Entry-Level Positions in Foodservice Systems Management. Chicago, The American Dietetic Association, 1983.

**Spears, Marian.: The First Year of a Coordinated Undergraduate Program in Foodsystems Management. *J. Am. Diet. Assoc.* 62:417, 1973.

The education required includes entry–level qualifications with three or less years of experience. Specific areas of study include:

—Principles of Food Systems Management

Provides an overall view of the management of food systems, including personnel involved in food preparation and service; equipment for operation; the purchasing of food and supplies; and the management of time and money.

—Quantity food purchasing and preparation

Provides indepth experience in menu planning, food preparation techniques and cooking procedures to assure quality food production.

—Development, utilization and maintenance of physical resources

Provides education in planning a food service facility, with exposure to equipment salesmen, consultants, engineers, and architects in developing the layout plan. Learns how to write equipment specifications and prepare cost estimates. Also, equipment operation, sanitation and preventive maintenance guidelines.

—Operations Analysis

Knowledge is gained in computer programming for use as a decision–making tool in food service for cost containment, food purchasing, stock maintenance, and as a carryover into clinical dietetics for modified diet menu planning and preparation.

Job satisfaction is high when the administrative dietitian is able to assume several roles. These include (a) a middle–management role as the director of a foodservice system; (b) an advisor role to top–level administrators of the organization; and (c) as a personnel administrator of other dietitians, foodservice employees, and dietetic students.

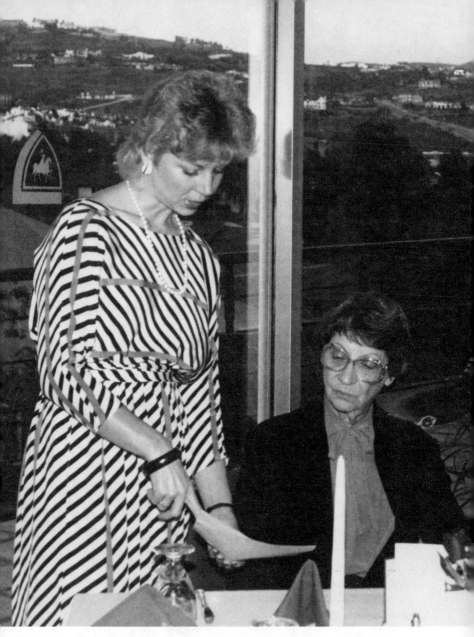

Terri Fields, R.D., works at a spa where she oversees a menu that is calorie controlled, low fat, contains no added salt and no sugar. Photo: Canyon Ranch Resort.

Barriers to career development and expansion in this area include (a) lack of visability; (b) the perception that dietitians, in general, lack adequate management skills; and (c) the actual shortage of dietitians willing to assume management positions, which causes hospital and other administrators to look elsewhere to hire administrative personnel.

Current and future technology will aide in the development of new administrative roles and challenges. The administrative dietitian must be willing to sacrifice traditional approaches and adopt new methods to deal with cost containment, while maintaining quality foodservice, increased productivity, and an increase in food and clinical nutrition services. To meet these challenges, the administrative dietitian must be assertive, knowledgeable, have the desire to work long and hard hours, and be "goals–oriented."

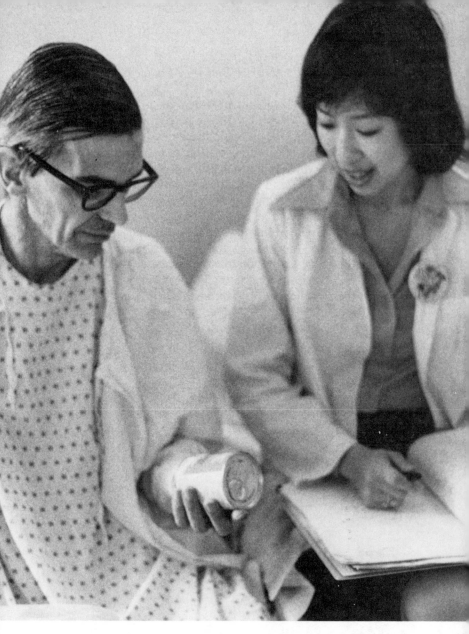

In a hospital setting a dietitian may be part of a team of professionals that includes a physician, pharmicist, nurse, and others to provide total health care to a patient. Photo: University of Chicago Medical Center.

CHAPTER 8

THE DIETITIAN AND OTHER HEALTH PROFESSIONALS

A professional is defined as an individual engaged in a field requiring specialized knowledge and often long and intensive academic preparation."* As a professional, the dietitian may interact with other professionals in order to provide the best care possible to the client. The team members may include a physician, pharmacist, exercise physiologist, nurse, psychologist, and others. The potential role of each will be discussed here.

One example of a team practice environment would concern the treatment of obesity. Obesity therapy requires psychological, medical, physical fitness, and dietary management. The concept of the team approach is imperative for the successful treatment of this problem and others. In this approach, the dietitian, as the primary care provider, may be responsible for medical monitoring, behavioral and cognitive counseling, and nutrition education. The dietitian may also be responsible for the patient's total care and may act as the coordinator of all team efforts. In this example, the

---

*Webster's Ninth New Collegiate Dictionary, (1983), s.v. "professional."

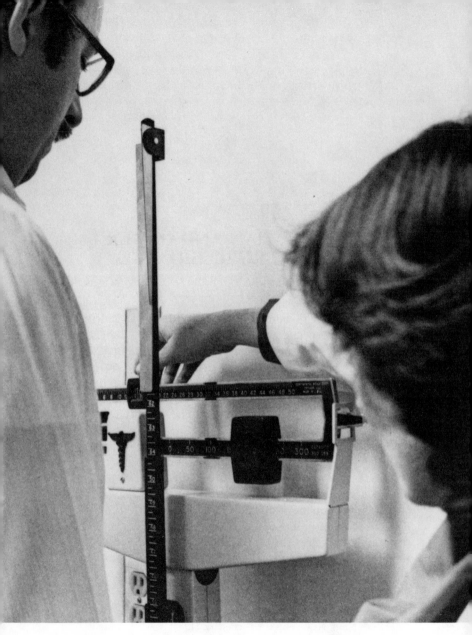

In monitoring a patient's progress the dietitian may take blood pressure, weigh the patient weekly, and order lab tests. Photo: Thomas Davis Clinic.

dietitian requires medical and psychological training, as well as traditional dietetic experience.

The medical role of the dietitian may be to take blood pressure, weigh the patient weekly, and order appropriate lab tests. As she or he monitors these aspects, problems can be related to the physician to assure complete medical care. The dietitian may also arrange an appointment with an exercise physiologist for a fitness evaluation and initiate an exercise program.

It is important for the dietitian to develop a relationship with the patient so that personal problems can be discussed. Basic counseling techniques may be used to help patients to better understand their behavior. The dietitian may also be qualified to identify more serious psychological problems, and refer the patient to a psychologist or psychiatrist in the community.*

This example of the team concept depicts how the dietitian may work closely with allied health professionals to provide "total care" to the patient. Other ways in which the dietitian may interact with allied health professionals include:

- —Consultation with a pharmacist to discuss drug–nutrient interaction, vitamin/mineral supplementation, or parenteral/enteral product use.
- —Interaction with a nurse to attain information regarding actual patient progress, and home health care problems.

As a professional working with other health team members, the dietitian must be confident, knowledgeable, and be able to apply all acquired skills to provide treatment to patients and to effectively communicate with other professionals.

---

*Anne Fletcher, R.D., "The Nutritionist as the Primary Care Provider in a Team Approach to Obesity", *The American Dietitian Association*, 80:253, March, 1982.

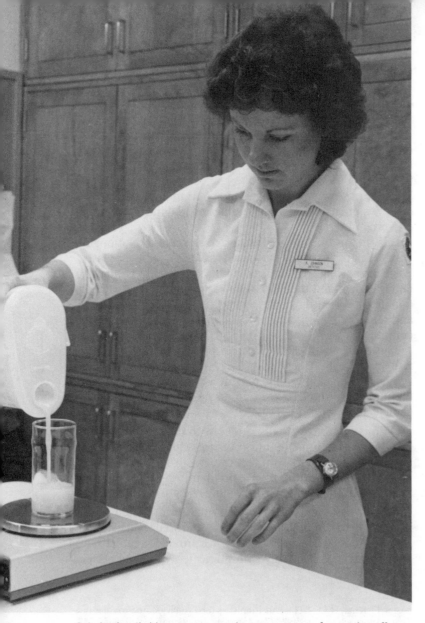

Salaries for dietitians vary across the country, some factors that affect salary range for an entry level position are, area of specialty and location of practice. Photo: Saint Mary's Hospital, Rochester, Minnesota.

CHAPTER 9

SALARIES AND JOB SATISFACTION

SALARIES

It is important to realize that salary levels for dietitians vary greatly. Some of the variables which would affect salary range include: practice specialty, area of the nation, size of the city, length of employment, experience, practice environment, the number of qualified professionals in the area, the cost of living, and others. National salary comparisons are scarce. The American Dietetic Association in 1981 reported that the median salary of experienced clinical dietitians for the United States as a whole was $18,000. With median salaries ranging from a low of $17,300 in the Southwest to a high of $19,800 in the West.*

Another survey completed in October, 1981 by the Bureau of Labor Statistics documented earnings of hospital dietitians by city.** They reported the following incomes:

---

*William W. Baldyga. Results From The 1981 Census of The American Dietetic Association. *J. Am. Diet. Assoc.* 83:343, 1983.
**Salaries and Benefits of Dietetic Personnel. *J. Am. Diet. Assoc.* 82:417, 1983.

Atlanta	$17,056
Chicago	$18,491
Cleveland	$19,739
Denver	$21,258
Detroit	$21,882
Kansas City	$18,387
Los Angeles	$21,008
Miami	$18,013
Milwaukee	$19,947
Minneapolis	$19,032
Portland	$20,758
San Francisco	$24,211
Seattle	$19,282

In a more recent survey conducted in Tucson, Arizona in March, 1985 the salary ranges for hospital dietitians were compared. These starting salary ranges combined from four hospitals are represented below.

	Median
Registered Dietitian, Level I	$18,980
Registered Dietitian, Level II	$21,262
Registered Dietitian, Specialty area	$24,003

Level I is defined as a registered dietitian with a Bachelor of Science degree with limited experience. Level II is defined as a registered dietitian with one to two years of experience with a Bachelor's or Master's of Science degree. The Specialty R.D. category considers expertise in a specific area, i.e., a Renal Center or Cardiac Rehabilitation Center.

The 1985 salary levels reported in Tucson represent an 18 percent increase in salary levels for experienced dietitians when compared to the median salary ranges for dietitians in the United States as a whole, reported in 1981.

Other areas of compensation which should be valued, when considering positions are Employee Benefits.* These benefits are a valuable asset to the nutrition professional. These additional benefits may include:

1. Disability benefits, sick and mental health leave; insurance—group life, accident, hospitalization; other:
   - 12-day sick leave per year
   - group life insurance equal to annual salary, hospitalization and medical insurance
   - dental insurance
   - discounts on goods and services purchased from company
   - employee meals
   - profit sharing
   - special bonuses
2. Vacation and holidays
3. Plan for salary increments and opportunities for advancement
4. Retirement Plans
5. Professional growth, i.e., for attendance at professional meetings, education, sabbaticals
6. Travel allowances
7. Employee fitness program and facility.

It is obvious that minimum salary levels have increased since 1981 and the available data limited to Tucson for 1985 is inadequate to represent the salary levels now available. However, as a perspective nutrition professional it is important to check with area practice groups about current salaries and benefits. Another resource is the classified ad section of the journal of The American Dietetic Association. This sec-

---

*Position Paper on Recommended Salaries and Employment Practies for Members of The American Dietetic Association. *J. Am. Diet. Assoc.* 78:62, 1981.

tion will provide regional salaries for current openings in the field and the qualifications necessary.

JOB SATISFACTION

In today's ever expanding and changing job market it is becoming more important to choose a career that will provide stimulation and rewards. Nutrition seems to be one of these career choices.

In a study which looked at work–related values among professions in dietetic services the findings attributed job satisfaction primarily to satisfaction with the work itself and supervision, with pay and with co–workers. This study also reported a high level of satisfaction among dietitians as a group. Dietitians responding to a general question on satisfaction with their position, showed that thirty-nine (39) percent were well satisfied and forty–three (43) percent were satisfied.*

Another study surveyed dietitians and asked "If you had to do it over again, would you make the same career choice." Sixty–five (65) percent of the sample indicated that they would make the same career choice.**

There are multiple aspects of a job which lead to job satisfaction. These have been summarized by Loche, who feels that the values or conditions most conducive to job satisfaction are: (1) mentally challenging work with which an individual can cope successfully; (2) personal interest in the

---

*Calbeck, Doris; Vaden, Allene and Richard Vaden. Work-Related Values and Satisfactions. *J. Am. Diet. Assoc.* 75:434, 1979.
**Aguesti-Johnson, Clair and Elizabeth Miles. Role Ambiguity, Role Conflict, and Job Satisfaction of Dietitians. *J. Am. Diet. Assoc.* 81:559, 1982.

work: (3) work which is not too physically tiring; (4) rewards for performance which are just, informative and in line with physical needs and which facilitate accomplishment of work goals; (6) high self–esteem; and (7) agents in the work place who help the employee attain job values such as interesting work, pay and promotions, whose basic values are similar to the employees' and who minimize role conflict and ambiguity.* **

Finally, it is important for the nutrition professional to evaluate all aspects of the potential job to determine if the employer can provide the satisfying work environment and work experience for the development of a rewarding career. The time has come when the professionals must determine whether they are "right" for the job and whether they can enthusiastically tackle the job expectations to achieve job satisfaction.

---

*Loche, E. A. The Nature and Causes of Job Satisfaction, in Dunnette M. (ed): *Handbook of Industrial Psychology and Organization Behavior.* Chicago, Rand McNally, 1976.
**Broski, David and Sandy Cook. The Job Satisfaction of Allied Health Professionals. *J. Allied Health.* Fall 1978, p. 282.

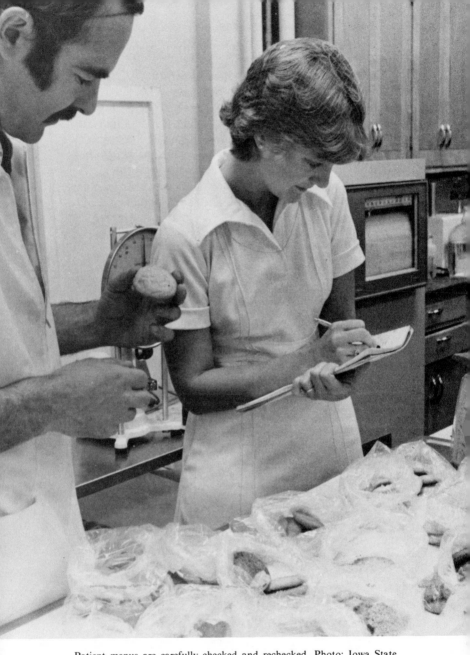

Patient menus are carefully checked and rechecked. Photo: Iowa State University.

CHAPTER 10

THE DIETETIC TECHNICIAN—
A SUPPORTIVE
NUTRITION POSITION

It is generally recognized that dietitians need assistance in performance of their professional responsibilities. Dietetic Technicians are technically skilled individuals who have been prepared to assume a supportive nutrition role and work under the guidance of a registered dietitian.*

The registered dietitian oversees the assessment, planning, and evaluation of individual patients with a dietetic technician assisting in any or all phases of the nutrition care process. The dietetic technician has responsibilities in assigned areas of nutrition care; such as, dietary instruction of selected individuals, consultation with the health team and monitoring of patient food quality and acceptance.

The American Dietetic Association recognizes these roles as appropriate for the dietetic technician who has completed an approved associate degree program.

At the "client" level, the clinical dietetic technician assists the registered dietitian in clinical practice to provide direct nutrition services to patients. The technician is responsible for:

---

*Position Papers in Clinical Dietetics. *J. Am. Diet. Assoc.* 80:256, 1982.

1. Using predetermined criteria in screening patients to identify those at nutritional risk and collecting data for use in assessing dietary status.
2. Following guidelines established by the registered dietitian to develop nutrition care plans for individual patients.
3. Providing technical services in the implementation of nutrition care plans.
4. Monitoring the effect of nutrition intervention and assessing patient food acceptance.
5. Providing diet counseling and education to individuals not at nutritional risk.

Within the second level, "intra–professional" relationships, the dietetic technician cooperates with the clinical dietitian in promoting standards of practice and using current knowlege to solve nutrition problems of individual patients.

At the third or "inter–professional" level, the technician is responsible for coordinating the nutrition care of assigned patients with other health services, and coordinating designated nutrition care plans with institutional food service activities.

At the "intra–organizational" level the dietetic technician utilizes established standards and procedures to implement the system of patient nutrition care. This responsibility includes:

1. Utilizing established procedures for making available designated special food products and dietary supplements.
2. Supervising diet clerks and other patient food service personnel.
3. Developing and implementing a program of orientation, training, and inservice education for patient food service personnel.

Employment environments for the dietetic technicial include community hospitals, intermediate or skilled nursing facilities or university medical centers. This indicates that health care is the primary employment outlet.*

Like the registered dietitian specializing in specific areas, the dietetic technician is expanding into sub-specialty areas. These sub-specialties may include work in:

— **Clinical Psychiatric Areas**

This specialty requires additional training in psychiatry, dealing with aggressive behavior, small group dynamics, care of the elderly, drug/food interaction, and diet and heart disease/hypertension.

— **Pediatric Practice**

This sub-specialty will expand the dietetic technician's role into assessment of maternal and child health, research and patient education.**

— **Critical Care**

Expanded roles may include increased patient contact to determine likes and dislikes and increased communication with food service for development of food formulas for the critically ill patient.

DIETETIC TECHNICIAN EDUCATION

The dietetic technician is a professional who holds an associate of arts degree and has completed 450 hours of supervised experience in the area of either nutritional care

---

*Simonis, Patricia, et. al.: Dietetic Technician's Performance: Supervisory and Self-Assessments. *J. Am. Diet. Assoc.* 82:271, 1983.
**Meyering, Suzanne.: An Exploratory Study of Trends in Specialities in Clinical Dietetics. June, 1981.

or foodservice management. The technician is viewed as the assistant to the clinical dietitian or the public health nutritionist. The approved program of dietetic technician education prepares the technician to conduct patient interviews; to assist patients in the daily choice of a balanced diet; to give routine dietary instructions; to arrange meal plans for modified diets; to assist patients in health care institutions or clients in the community in meal planning and food purchasing for the entire family; and to assist the dietitian or nutritionist in preparing educational materials for various teaching programs.*

The table below represents the recommended American Dietetic Association pattern for an approved program of dietetic technician education leading to competency in nutrition care.**

In *Nutrition Care I* students study normal nutrition. This course covers: why and how people eat; what influences malnutrition; how to bring about changes in food habits; cultural food patterns; the nature of food and its work in the body; the normal process of digestion, absorption, and metabolism; nutrients and their functions; nutrition in the life cycle; and food fads.

Nutrition Care II covers the study of diet therapy. This course is concerned with the nutritional care of the patient with problems of the upper gastrointestinal region and progresses to nutritional care of the patient with congestive heart failure, hypertension, atherosclerosis, hyperlipoproteinemea, obesity and diabetes.

---

*Doherty, Elizabeth, R.D.: Educating the Dietetic Technician. *J. Am. Diet. Assoc.* 62:421, 1973.
**Essentials of an Acceptable Program of Dietetic Technician Education.* *Revised.* Chicago: Am. Diet. Assn., 1971.

Course	Semester Hours
Semester 1	
Nutrition Care I	3
Supervised Field Experience	1
Foods	3
Health Field	1
Contemporary Sociology	3
Open Course	3
Open Course	3
Total	17
Semester 2	
Nutrition Care II	3
Supervised Field Experience	2
Education	3
Health Field	1
Open Course	3
Open Course	3
Total	15
Semester 3	
Nutrition Care III	3
Supervised Field Experience	3
Health Care Delivery System	3
Management	3
Open Course	3
Total	15
Semester 4	
Nutrition Care IV	3
Supervised Field Experience	4
Dietetic Seminar	1
Open Course	3
Open Course	3
Open Course	3
Total	17

Nutrition Care III involves study of the general problems of nutritional care of patients with problems of (a) digestion, absorption, and metabolism and (b) fluid and electrolyte balance.

Nutrition Care IV emphasizes community nutrition learning to deal with inborn errors of metabolism, anemias, arthritis and more.

The *Foods* course considers an overview of food; the Basic four food groups; principles of menu planning and food purchasing for the home, including budgeting; food stamps; and interpretation of food advertising and labels. It also covers food additives, food sanitation and spoilage, unit pricing and FDA rulings.

Dietetic Orientation introduces the health field and the roles of practitioners in dietetics. The student is also introduced to various feeding systems and the team efforts to provide adequate nutrition care.

THE FUTURE

The future of employment as a dietetic technician is expanding as the increased utilization of the technician by various organizations will lead to cost containment, better use of supportive personnel, reduction in manpower needs, and functioning of dietitians at the level of proficiency for which they were educated.*

---

*Noland, M. S., and Steinberg, R.: Activities of Therapeutic Dietitians—A Survey Report. *J. Am. Diet. Assoc.* 46:477, 1965.

Lunsden, J. E., Zolker, K., Strutz, P., Moore, S. T., Sanchez, A., and Abbey, D.: Delegation of Functions by Dietitians to Dietetic Technicians. *J. Am. Diet. Assoc.* 69:143, 1976.

Beck, E.: "Utilization of Dietetic Technicians in Hospitals." Unpublished master's theses, Loma Linda University, 1978.

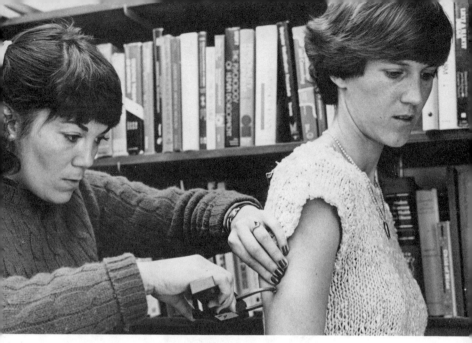

Dietitions and technicians will assist clients by monitoring their response to diet modifications. Photo: University of Arizona Health Sciences Center.

Rose, J. C., Zolker, K., Vyhmeister, I., Abbey, D., and Burke, I.: Performance of Task Functions by American Dietetic Association Dietetic Technicians. *J. Am. Diet. Assoc.* 76:563, 1980.

Hubbard, R. M. I., and Donaldson, B.: Estimating Professional Manpower Needs for Hospital Dietary Departments. *J. Am. Diet. Assoc.* 53:211, 1968.

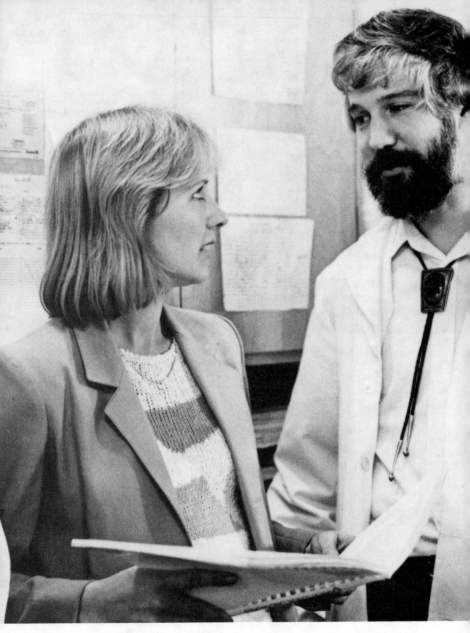

Need for dietitians is expected to increase in private industry and non-institutional health care facilities, more than in hospitals and higher education. Photo: Park West Clinic.

CHAPTER 11

"NETWORKING SUCCESS: DESIGN FOR TOMORROW"

The subject of nutrition* has never been as popular as it is now. The general public is increasing its interest in health from a wellness standpoint. These facts help create a positive environment for the practice of dietetics.

On the other hand, many dietitian's positions may be threatened. Encroachment by other professions in the areas of nutrition and dietetics, increasing numbers of health gurus, deregulation by the federal government, the cost–containment mandate in health care, and slow–to–change educational institutions all threaten the dietitians' current practice.**

The practice environment is changing, however. Dietitians willing to change and grow, to study hard, to keep up to date, and to choose the profession as a lifelong career will find the challenges can be met and a bright future is possible.

---

*Young, Eleanor A. Nutrition: An Integral Aspect of Medical Education. *J. Am. Diet. Assoc.* 82:482, 1983.
**Watson, Donna R. President's Page: Challenges Facing the Dietetic Profession. *J. Am. Diet. Assoc.* 84:1484, 1984.

THE CHANGING SCENE

Six factors influence the demand for dietetic services. These include: 1) socioeconomic trends; 2) public policy; 3) health values, attitudes, and behaviors; 4) technology diffusion; 5) competition; and 6) changes in the profession.*

1. Social and economic trends are influenced by:
   a. Population demographics which affect the supply of professionals, the needs for goods and services, and the location of clients.
   b. The economic climate which affects public funding for nutrition programs, the ability of clients to pay for the services, food pricing and the supply of professionals.
   c. Health expenditures which affect available dollars for preventive services and reimbursement policies.
2. Public policy is influenced by:
   a. The existence of publicly supported nutrition and food programs.
   b. The degree of regulatory control.
   c. Reimbursement schedules.
   d. Wage guidelines.
3. Health values, attitudes, and behaviors are influenced by:
   a. The population's attitudes toward nutrition services and care.
   b. Consumer oriented decisions regarding health care.
   c. Payment for nutrition services.
4. Technological advances influence:
   a. The delivery of food and services.
   b. The use of communication resources and computer applications

---

*Fitz, Polly A., et. al. Demand for Dietitians: Taking Control of the Future. *J. Am. Diet. Assoc.* 83:68, 1983.

c. Creation of new dietetic roles.
5. Competition influences:
   a. The consumers' ability to seek the dietitian for nutrition care.
   b. The fees for services and the payment system.
6. Changes in the profession influence:
   a. The visibility of the dietitian.
   b. The supply of dietitians.
   c. The demand for nutrition services.

The influence of these six areas will continue to change practice environments and expand the nutrition services requested by industry, government and the general public.

The direction of the future demand for dietitians based on the above listed influences on the profession is presented below. This represents the optimal scenario for future demand based on employer type.

EMPLOYER	OPTIMAL SCENARIO
Non-government Organization	
Health care facilities/organizations	Increase
Educational institutions	No Change
Commercial	Increase
Other (church, non-profit, etc.)	No Change
Government	
"City or County"	
Health care facilities/organizations	Increase
Educational institutions	No Change
State	
Health care facilities/organizations	Increase
Educational institutions	No Change

Federal
  Health care facilities/organizations   Increase
  Educational institutions   No Change

Solo or Partnership   Increase
Dietitians or other health providers
(M.D., D.M.D., etc.)   Increase

This scenario contains a mixture of positive and negative elements. Fewer registered dietitians will be employed in hospitals, in higher education and by government; while more will have jobs in private industry, consulting practices and non–institutional health care facilities.

What impact will this changing scenario have on dietetic practice?

The dietetic practitioner will have to be aware and progress in five major areas. These areas include:

1. Professional Education.
2. Research.
3. Marketing of Nutrition and Services.
4. Cost–effective Health Care.
5. The American Dietetic Association.

EDUCATION

New competencies or enhancement of current competencies will be demanded as dietitians move into advanced levels of practice. The only way other professionals will recognize your expertise is for you to demonstrate that you have the knowledge and the competency in specific skills to perform specific tasks.

For the *Clinical Dietitian Specialist,* the need will be for additional competency in biochemistry, pathophysiology, pharmacology, management (including cost/benefit analysis), computer applications to nutritional care, development of leadership skills for influencing legislation in the political arena, and professional assertiveness.

For the *Administrative Dietitian,* the need will be for competencies in cost/benefit analysis, computer applications to food service management, cooperative group purchasing, enhanced writing skills for technical and administrative reports, and development of leadership skills for influencing legislation in the political arena.

For the *Community Dietitian,* the need will be for increased emphasis on leadership for "wellness" programs and lifestyle change clinics and programs, an understanding of the cultural values and food habits of ethnic groups, and development of skills needed for writing grant proposals.*

RESEARCH

Research is becoming an essential component to document the value of nutrition services and for achieving third-party payment for services provided. Therefore, it is essential for the dietetic practitioner to develop consistent care, based on standardized protocols or criteria which have been developed for quality assurance.

Clinical, community, and administrative dietitians must be able to justify their services by documentation of both process and outcome. The model below represents the process of nutritional counseling leading to economic benefits, an area in which research is needed.

---

*Zolber, Kathleen. The President's Page. *J. Am. Diet. Assoc.* 81:594, 1982.

MODEL*

Nutritional	Changes in	Altered	
Counseling	→ Food Intake	→ Risk Factors	→

Desirable Health	Economic	
Outcomes	→ Benefits.	

The desired outcome of research will be to clearly demonstrate that nutrition services contribute to the quality of life and can be provided cost-effectively.

MARKETING

Many consumers are not informed about nutrition services which are available to them, or about dietitians who are qualified to provide the services. Individuals depend upon physicians and other allied health professionals to advise them about health and nutrition services. Because these professionals are not well informed about the range of nutrition services which are available, referrals are often limited.**

The dietitian must, therefore, apply marketing strategies to inform the public and other health care providers about the nutrition services available and that the dietitian is the professional educated to provide these nutrition services.

Target groups of this marketing effort should include the general public, third-party payers, specific employer and

---

*Mason, Marion, Ph.D., R. D., et. al. Requisites of Advocacy: Philosophy, Research, Documentation. Phase II of the Costs and Benefits of Nutritional Care. *J. Am. Diet. Assoc.* 80:213, 1982.

**Haschke, Marilyn. President's Page: Marketing in Dietetics. *J. Am. Diet. Assoc.* 84:934, 1984.

employee groups and public policy makers.* In addition, the current emphasis on wellness will increase the roles of the dietitian and will expand marketing of professional services, especially in preventive counseling to industry and to the public directly.

PROVISION OF COST-EFFECTIVE HEALTH CARE

Predictions for health care, in general, indicate a continued growth of alternate delivery systems, such as health maintenance organizations (HMOs). Services traditionally provided in hospitals will continue to be converted to out-of-hospital care by provision of lower levels of care in skilled nursing facilities and home health care. Corporate control of health care will continue to grow. Support of employers for employee health promotion will continue through growing numbers of wellness programs. Consumers are becoming very cost conscious and will seek quality services at a reasonable cost.**

The nature of these changes which are now taking place in health care is so fundamental as to present a threat to those who fail to respond and an opportunity to those who take action promptly.

Action by dietetic practitioners is the key. There is a need again to market nutrition services to the general public, employer/employee groups, third-party payers, prepaid health plans, and national and state public policy formulators.

Dietitians will be required to be more creative than ever before to solve the problems that practitioners face. Dietitians must demonstrate the value of their services by documenting the cost and the effectiveness of services.

---

*Haschke, Marilyn. President's Page: The Potential of the Association: A Dynamic Balance of Management. *J. Am. Diet. Assoc.* 84:689, 1984.
**Haschke, Marilyn. President's Page: DRG's: Impact and Implications for Action. *J. Am. Diet. Assoc.* 83:584, 1983.

As competition increases to provide cost–effective health care, the dietitian must take control of providing nutrition services as physicians, nurses, and pharmacists increase the delivery of nutrition services as part of their practice.

THE AMERICAN DIETETIC ASSOCIATION

The Association provides a means for the dietetic profession to identify those issues that must be addressed, to set goals that need to be accomplished, and to conduct programs that will strengthen the ability of dietitians to meet the needs of society. In doing so, the Association supports the profession by enabling members to work together to achieve vital goals which are unattainable by individual efforts.

In addition, the Association provides essential communication for members via:

- The Journal
- The Courier and other media and publications.
- Providing information on topics ranging from legislation, public relations, dietetic education, etc.
- Providing data and information about specific areas of practice.

The challenge to survive has become a joint responsibility. The dietitian working with The American Dietetic Association through dietetic practice groups and state and district associations must assert her/him–self and must work within The Code of Ethics and By–Laws established by The American Dietetic Association. It is this joint effort which will allow the previous mentioned goals to be achieved.

CONCLUSION

To quote John Naisbitt in his book, *The Year Ahead: 1985,* he states: "The Health industry is booming, creating jobs not only for nurses, but also for dietitians. . . . In fact, the number of dietitians has grown from fewer than 35,000 in 1971 to more than 60,000 in 1982."*

It *is* an exciting time to be and become a nutrition professional.

---

*Naisbitt, John: *The Year Ahead: 1985.* The Naisbitt Group, New York, New York. 1984.

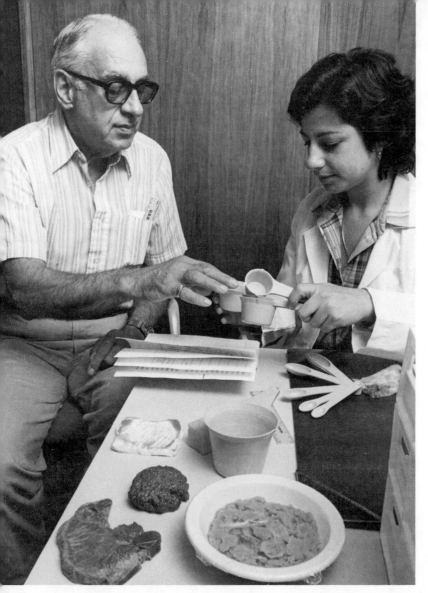

Dietitians in public health are usually employed by health agencies at the federal, state, and local levels. They often specialize in work for a particular segment of the population, whether it be a geographical or age group. Above, a nutritionist at the Human Nutrition Research Center on Aging explains the principles of a balanced diet to a volunteer subject. Photo: USDA.

CHAPTER 12

THE NATURE OF PUBLIC HEALTH/NUTRITION EDUCATION TODAY

PUBLIC HEALTH

Public Health Nutrition* is defined as population–based program planning, implementation, and evaluation in a health agency to improve the nutritional well–being of a population that may be defined geographically or categorically, i.e., children or pregnant women. The nutritional personnel are employed by health agencies at the federal, state and local levels; they conduct needs assessments to establish priorities for nutrition programs. Dietitians develop strategies for developing nutrition services; they implement the programs, evaluate them and revise, and establish new objectives.

Beginning in the mid 1960's, public health agencies increased direct nutrition services to populations at nutrition risk or with demonstrated nutrition needs as pregnant women, infants, and children. Services expanded so that by 1980 approximately one half of the nutrition personnel in local

---

*Dodds, Janic. Graduate Programs of Public Health Nutrition. *J. Am. Diet. Assoc.* 81:717, 1982.

health agencies were implementing WIC (Supplemental Food Program for Women, Infants and Children), a direct service program. The federal WIC program is designed to establish a clear relation between nutrition and health care services "to serve as an adjunct to good health care during critical times of growth and development."* ** The purpose of the program was to provide timely pre-natal care to reduce the incidence of low-birth weight infants.

There is a growing need in Public Health Nutrition professionals, at the federal level, there has been no sense of priorities of clear focus in maternal nutrition. Therefore, there are opportunities for professionals to become involved in program development and implementation, along with nutrition research. Research is needed to establish baseline data on the nutrition and health status of the public with special attention to infants, children and the elderly. At the same time, developing plans for the assessment of remaining vulnerable groups such as adolescents, pregnant women, the handicapped and the unemployed.

Also, community health centers, migrant health programs and the expansion of "primary health care" have established additional work environments for the Public Health Dietitian. These work environments include directing nutrition in state and local health departments with ampulatory clients in prevention and treatment centers.

NUTRITION EDUCATION

This area of nutrition specialty provides many work environment opportunities. The two to be discussed here include

---

*Jacobson, H. N. Nutrition and pregnancy. *J. Am. Diet. Assoc.* 60:26, 1972.
**Jacobson, H. N. Maternal Nutrition in the 1980's. *J. Am. Diet. Assoc.* 80:216, 1982.

nutrition education in the public school system and nutrition education in a fitness/health promotion program. Nutrition education in the school system may involve working for the government at the state level to expand nutrition programs or with city school districts. To work in this area four essential categories of expertise are important. These include:

(1) Nutrition and Food
   - to provide nutrition information to individuals and groups involved in education program development
   - To use knowledge about school food service to conduct nutrition related education programs
(2) Education
   - to work with teachers and food service personnel to implement and evaluate
(3) Communications
   - to use various media (video, audio, radio) as an integral part of a nutrition education program
(4) Government
   - To use the understanding about political processes as it relates to schools food programs

This area of nutrition specialty has progressed slowly. One of the main reasons is because government policies and programs change as administrations change and therefore funding available changes. However, the need for qualified professionals is rising and documented by the recommendation of the White House Conference of Food, Nutrition and Health: the need for a comprehensive and sequential program of nutrition education in U.S. schools.*

A second area of nutrition education involves health promotion programs. Personal efforts to overcome smoking

---

*Poolton, Martha. What Does the Nutrition Education Specialist Need to Know? *J. Nutri. Ed.* 9:105, 1977.

habits, alcohol and drug abuse, dietary excess, stress and physical inactivity are evidence of the new health awareness in this country.* As corporate America commits more resources to employee health promotion programs, due to their cost–effectiveness, more and more openings will become available for nutrition professionals to direct behavioral change programs.

The nutrition educator's roles in fitness/health promotion program may include:

- use of computer programs for nutrient analysis
- interviewing to obtain diet histories
- interpretation of biochemical tests
- percent body fat calculation and interpretation
- evaluation of nutritional status
- patient counseling to determine goals
- development of tools for recording patient progress and maintaining documentation for research
- group counseling and education
- development of posters and pamplets to use as education materials
- development of workshops to deal with behavior change, cooking techniques, restaurant eating and holidays, etc.
- writing for lay publications

These roles may vary depending on the actual work environment, however, they are all important for any health promotion program.

The educational preparation necessary would include a B.S. or M.S. degree in nutrition with minor course in exercise physiology or another related field, i.e., psychology, counseling, business administration, marketing. Also, status as an R.D. is important when competing for job openings. The

---

*White, P. L. and Selvey, N. Nutrition and the new health awareness. *JAMA* 247:2914, 1982.

more general knowledge and skill areas which should be acquired are:*

Dietetic Curriculum Applicable to a Fitness Program

Diadactic
Health risk analysis (health hazard appraisal) dealing with the risk of cardiovascular disease, diabetes, obesity, hypertension and poor eating habits.

Nutrition as it relates to exercise physiology

Nutrition and the athlete—current fads and practices

Skills
Nutrition assessment
- interviewing adapted to needs
- interpretation of anthropometric measurements body (fat) composition as influenced by exercise
- use and interpretation of computerized nutrient data
- calculation of risk based on health risk analysis
- generation of record system compatible with existing document systems
- counseling/follow-up while in co-participant role
- preparation/delivery of brief messages for impact in action-oriented setting
- written communication through newsletters/audio-visuals
- workshop planning and presentation based on group health needs and concerns
- Relationships with non-traditional health team (i.e., exercise physiologists)
- promotion of dietitian's role in fitness programs
- sharing expertise: providing and participating

---

*Wagstaff, M. and Mattfeldt-Beman, M. The fitness opportunity for dietetic educators and practitioners. *J. Am. Diet. Assoc.* 84:1465, 1984.

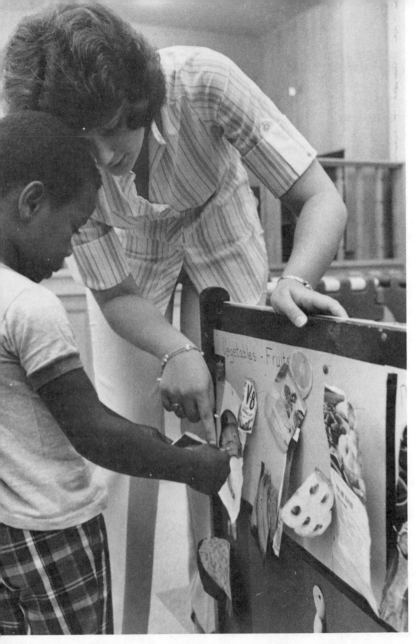
A dietitian works with a student in the classroom. Photo: Iowa State University.

The area of Public Health Nutrition and Nutrition Education are providing constant stimulation due to the diversity of work environments and work situations. For the dietitian not interested in the "traditional" clinical nutrition approach, these areas will continue to grow and challenge the nutrition professional to implement new ideas and programs.

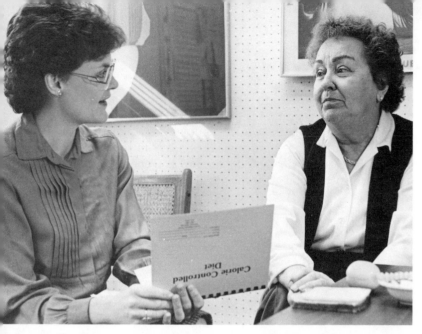

Two areas that the Registered Dietian may enter are private practice, above, and institutional health centers, below. Photo: Above, Associates in Professional Nutrition Counseling; below, University of Arizona Health Sciences Center.

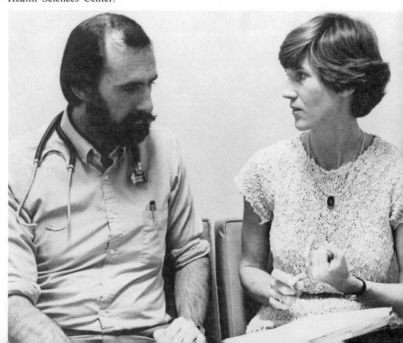

CHAPTER 13

INTERVIEWS WITH CURRENT PRACTITIONERS

Professionals, educators, counselors and others involved in the field of nutrition often forget how large the field of nutrition really is. Nutrition continues to be a rapidly growing discipline ranging in content from agriculture and animal sciences to human medicine. Because of our own particular interests, training and experience, each person in the field tends to see only a small portion of the full spectrum of nutrition. In an attempt to provide the interested student with as broad a spectrum as possible we have interviewed dietitians who are currently practicing. These interviews follow. They discuss 1) the current work environments and work roles 2) the education pathway followed 3) previous work experience and 4) the future.

NUTRITION CONSULTANT

Gail A. Levey, M.S., R.D.

Gail currently specializes in nutritional communication. She also is a writer, and contributes articles to major magazines, including *Health, Good Food, Weight Watchers, Video Reviews* and *Vegetarian Times.* She has researched articles for other writers, has written nutrition booklets, has discussed nutrition in the media, lectured, and consulted to businesses. Her undergraduate education was in Nutritional Sciences at Cornell University, and she completed her M.S. at Columbia University in Nutrition and Public Health. She then did a six-month work experience to become qualified to take the R.D. exam. She states "I realized the R.D. was essential."

Because there is a great variety of courses, and there is rapid change going on in the field, it is important for the future dietitian/nutritionist to review carefully the requirements of the areas in which he or she wishes to work, and to be sure to plan to meet those requirements.

Gail suggests that dietitians develop in the following areas if they expect to develop a varied practice.

- obtain a good nutrition/biochemistry education base
- acquire an advanced degree in a related area
- associate oneself with good mentors and peers
- time and travel flexibility is important
- need to keep up–to–date

To achieve career goals Gail states "It takes time, experience and persistence. Dietitians need to realize that there are a lot of innovative things to get into."

DIRECTOR OF DIETETIC EDUCATION PROGRAM: CENTRAL ARIZONA COMMUNITY COLLEGE

Elaine Kvitka, M.S., R.D.

Elaine is program director for a 2–year, 23–course diet technician program. This is a unique program because 14 of the 23 courses are available through PSI (Personalized System of Instruction). A student may enroll and receive packets of material for self instruction. The only criteria for admittance is that the students must have an R.D. advisor working with them. This program was developed for those individuals looking for a career in nutrition but who did not want a four-year degree.

Elaine received her B.S. degree from UCLA in Home Economics with a major emphasis in food and nutrition. While obtaining her M.S. degree she worked as a graduate assistant teaching lower division courses. In addition, she developed and taught an obesity control course. She wrote a job description for the position of Nutrition Consultant to the Student Health Center and got the job. She then taught at Ambassador College in Pasadena, California in Foods and Nutrition, where she wrote a textbook in meal management. She went on to become Training Coordinator for the Arizona Department of Health Services. She coordinated all nutrition education and training for 14 county and 10 tribal health programs throughout the state. She also provided 1) continuing education to nutrition professionals and para-professionals and 2) developed manuals, printed materials, and workshops, and maintained a library resource center.

In her career, Elaine has developed a broad and varied background of knowledge and skills, which has come about through working on several different kinds of programs, and also through writing and publishing.

Elaine feels the future nutrition professional must be assertive, creative, willing to take risks, and willing to do things differently. She states "There is tremendous expansion and opportunity in the field if we are willing to show what we have to offer by being creative and cost effective."

DIRECTOR OF NUTRITION, DIET AND FITNESS CENTER—GOOD HOUSEKEEPING INSTITUTE

Amy Barr, M.S., R.D.

Amy is involved with clearing all advertising which has anything to do with nutrition including food labeling, calorie content, nutrition claims and checking recipes. She also writes a column called "What's News: Nutrition, Diet and Fitness" for the Institute. In addition, she is involved in radio and TV tours which discuss current nutrition issues. The Center also provides the computer base software information on all the recipes published in the magazine. The Center currently employs one other dietitian, a home economist and a kitchen technician.

Amy received her B.S. in Home Economics with a major in Nutrition at the University of Nebraska, and completed an Ed.M. degree in nutrition at Tufts University, and an M.S. in Science Journalism at Boston University.

Amy relates that the hospital setting is not for everyone. Future job expansion includes nutrition positions in advertising, marketing, public relations and other areas of business. She feels that additional course work in business management, advertising, and communication is important for the future nutrition professional.

NUTRITIONIST/WRITER

Virginia Aronson, M.S., R.D.

Virginia is currently working as the Nutritionist/Writer for Harvard Department of Nutrition. She writes nutrition education materials for lay individuals and professionals. She has also written nine books and writes a monthly column for *Runners World* and *Shape Magazines.*

Her education began at the University of Vermont where she received her B.S. in Dietetics (a traditional program). She completed her Internship in New York and received her M.S. from Framingham State University in Nutrition with an emphasis in education. Following completion of her M.S. degree, she worked for the Community Health Education Department developing and implementing weight control clinics, group workshops and lectures.

Virginia feels that additional course work in education, writing, and communication and practice in working with media would be helpful to achieve a rewarding career. She perceives that a nutrition career will expand into 1) public education related areas, i.e., fitness centers 2) preventive/ wellness education and 3) nutrition writing and related communication.

MANAGER OF NUTRITION TECHNICAL SERVICES—GENERAL MILLS, INC.

Rita Warren, M.S., R.D.

Rita acts as the consultant for nutrition resources for internal groups within the company. Her department looks at the nutrition impact of products and nutrition labeling, and the department also discusses nutrition concerns with marketing. Other areas include providing nutrition education to health professionals via a newsletter, pamphlets and booklets, and providing nutrition education to schools. There are ten nutritionists employed by the department. All have at least the M.S. degree, and are R.D.'s or R.D.–qualified.

Rita received her undergraduate degree in Food Science with a minor in Chemistry, and her M.S. degree in Nutrition with a minor in Food Science. She worked in the Food

Chemistry lab at the University of Minnesota, then went to Pillsbury and worked on chemical analysis of foods.

Rita feels the skills which are important for future career development include knowledge about computers, communication, business, and an awareness about government nutrition policies.

TECHNICAL INFORMATION SPECIALIST
NATIONAL AGRICULTURAL LIBRARY

Carole Shore, M.S., R.D.

Carole has a unique position as a "librarian". There are only a few library staffs that she is aware of who have selected nutrition professionals and trained them in library management to provide nutrition–related services. Some of these are:

> The National Agricultural Library
> The Congressional-Research Service
> The National Medical Library

There are two major work areas. These include Acquisitions and Reference. Acquisitions deals with acquiring the selection of books, journals, and audio–visuals which the library will catalog. Reference Librarians are subject matter specialists who help clients receive the information they are interested in. They will also index, abstract material, and work with computers to provide short bibliographical data on nutrition topics. Carole currently works with three other Registered Dietitians.

Carole's educational background includes her B.S. in Dietetics following a traditional program with an Internship. Her M.S. degree was completed in Medical Dietetics at Ohio State University. Her previous work experience included research with the United States Department of Agriculture, developing United States Dietary Goals.

Carole feels the future nutrition student should choose a career which provides the potential to "ladder" or move upward in responsibility and authority. There is a need to combine two disciplines, i.e., Dietetics and Information Science; Dietetics and Management. She perceives growth potential in public health and community nutrition because of the increase in hospital costs and in the aging population. Also the information explosion will create a greater need in library sciences.

LECTURER/WRITER/CONSULTANT

Linda Houtkooper M.S., R.D.

As a lecturer Linda has taught undergraduate studies in nutrition–as–it–applies–to–life. This work involved organizing visual aides, writing lectures, and evaluating student projects and progress, and providing student counseling. As a writer Linda currently writes for *Swimming World Magazine* a monthly column on questions related to nutrition and swimming performance. She has also provided a year–long service of nutrition articles to the magazine. In addition to writing for lay publications, she has written for professional journals. A recent publication discussed training methods for implementing a nutrition–fitness curriculum in elementary schools. As a consultant, Linda has provided sports nutrition information to aerobic instructors' workshops, she has developed and implemented a nutrition weight management course for an employee fitness program and has done literature review/research to up–date paraprofessionals.

Linda has received her B.S. in Home Economic Education

with a minor in Guidance and Counseling. She is currently working toward her Ph.D. in Nutritional Sciences with a minor in Exercise Physiology. Her dissertation involves validation of new methods of analysis for body composition determination.

When asked about the future, Linda sees nutrition evolving in interdisciplinary areas. She foresees dietitians working with behavior therapists, exercise physiologists, pharmacists, and physicians, doing research and program development for the community, in business and industry, and at universities.

PROFESSOR/NUTRITIONIST
UNIVERSITY OF ARIZONA

Mary Ann Kight, Ph.D., R.D.

Mary Ann's current area of practice involves research, development, and education related to nutritional diagnosis in the practice of R.D.'s. She describes a traditional 4-step care process: *Assessment, Plan, Implementation* and *Evaluation.* She feels that for dietitians to reach a higher level of professionalism, an autonomous role or posture must be achieved. Therefore, a fifth level of care—the Diagnostic Step—previously performed solely by physicians, is now included in and defined as a role for the dietitian.

Dr. Kight's education background began with her B.S. in Human Nutrition and Dietetics; her M.S. and Ph.D. Degrees were in Biochemistry and Nutrition. She has remained in the academic environment to establish research and teaching credentials which she felt were prerequisite to the diagnostic contribution.

For the future, Dr. Kight states, "Through the teaching

of and use of the five–step–care process, diagnostic categories, nutritional diagnostic criteria, and nutritional diagnostic standards of practice, the R.D. will achieve an autonomous role. This will not be automatic. It will require strong continuing education programs followed by a stronger formal education."

CONCLUSION

It is exciting to learn about the variety of positions available for the Nutrition Professional. It is evident that career opportunities can provide a rewarding work environment and the ability to develop as a team member. Although a formalized education program, registration status, continuing education and a mentor/peer group seem to be all essential for the development of a Nutrition Professional.

GLOSSARY

Administrative Dietitian—a member of the management team who affects the nutritional care of groups through the management of food service systems that provide optimal nutrition and quality food.

American Dietetic Association, The—a professional organization responsible for establishing educational and supervised clinical experience requirements and standards of practice in dietetics.

Clinical Dietitian—a health care professional credentialed as a registered dietitian who affects the nutrition care of individuals and groups in health and illness. The clinical dietitian provides nutrition assessment, planning, implementation (including education and referral), and evaluation services; provides consultation for foodservice to coordinate nutrition care services, manages departmental and personnel functions for nutrition care services; delineates and manages external influences on the delivery of nutrition care. The clinical dietitian educates and coordinates activities as a member of the health care team; maintains skill and knowledge in optimal nutrition care; and conducts applied research.

Community Dietitian—a specialized dietetic professional

in a community setting who affects the nutrition services to individuals and groups in health and illness. The community dietitian provides nutrition assessment, planning, implementation (including education and referral) and evaluation services; plans, organizes, coordinates, and evaluates selected components of nutrition services for an organization. The community dietitian coordinates activities and educates, as a member of the team providing health care and/or nutrition services, and maintains skill and knowledge in optimal nutrition care.

Consultant Dietitian—has experience in administrative or clinical dietetic practice, affects the management of human effort and facilitates resources with advice or services in nutritional care.

Coordinated Undergraduate Dietetic Program—is a formalized baccalaureate educational program in dietetics sponsored by an accredited college or university and accredited by The American Dietetic Association. The curriculum is designed to coordinate didactic and supervised clinical experiences to meet the qualifications for practice in the profession of dietetics.

Dietetic Internship—is a formalized, post–baccalaureate educational program in dietetics sponsored and conducted by an organization and accredited by The American Dietetic Association. The curriculum of the program is designed to provide didactic and supervised clinical experience to meet the qualifications for practice in dietetics.

Dietetics—a profession concerned with the science and art of human nutritional care, an essential component of health science. It includes the extending and imparting of knowledge concerning foods which will provide nutrients sufficient for health and during disease throughout the life cycle, and the management of group feeding.

Dietetic Technician—a technically skilled person who has successfully completed an associate degree program which meets the educational standards established by The American Dietetic Association. The dietetic technician, working under guidance of an R.D., or an A.D.A. dietitian, has responsibilities in assigned areas in food service management, in teaching foods and nutrition principles, and in dietary counseling.

Dietetic traineeship—an individualized, post-baccalaureate educational program in dietetics sponsored by an organization and approved by The American Dietetic Association. Each program is designed to provide didactic and supervised clinical experiences to meet the qualifications for practice in the profession of dietetics.

Enteral Nutrition—chemically defined liquid diets delivered by mouth or tube feedings.

Entry-level—in each level of practice, position requiring the minimum level of training and experience; operationally defined as position which can be filled by a person with three years or less experience.

Foodservice System—an organized, integrated, or coordinated whole composed of diverse, but interrelated and interdependent parts, (e.g., menu planning, procurement, production, distribution, and service) for accomplishment of objectives.

Foodservice Systems Management—systems: an array of components formed into a unified whole to perform a systematic, purposeful activity. When used in conjunction with food service, it would be the components what make up the production and service of food. Management: the process of achieving desired results by the effective use of human effort and facilitating resources.

Health Care Team—a group of health care professionals who provide coordinated services to achieve optimal health care of the client.

Nutrition—the science of food, the nutrients and other substances therein, their action, interaction, and balance in relation to health and disease, and the processes by which the organism ingests, digests, absorbs, transports, utilizes, and excretes food substances. In addition nutrition must be concerned with social, economic, cultural, and psychologic implications of food and eating (definition of the Council on Foods and Nutrition, American Medical Association, 1963).

Nutritional Care—application of the science and art of human nutrition in helping people select and obtain food for the primary purpose of nourishing their bodies in health or disease throughout the life cycle. This participation may be in single or combined functions; in food service systems management of groups; in extending knowledge of food and nutrition principles through research; in teaching these principles for application according to particular situations; and in dietary counseling.

Nutrition Assessment—determination of nutrition status and history of the client (individual); determination of certain facts indicative of nutrition status and possible malnutrition of individuals (community).

Nutrition Care Plan—a detailed formulation of a program of action to meet the nutrition needs of clients.

Nutrition Status—the condition of physical health and well being of the body as related to the consumption and utilization of food for growth, maintenance and repair.

Parenteral Nutrition—any form of nutrient delivered by central or peripheral vein.

Public Health Nutritionist—the member of the public health agency staff with advanced training who takes the lead in assessing community nutrition needs, and plans, organizes, directs or coordinates, and evaluates the nutrition component of the health agency's services.

Registered Dietitian (R.D.®)—a person who has completed eligibility requirements (i.e., education and experience) and passed an examination of basic knowledge related to dietetic practice and who maintains competence through participation in approved continuing education.

Research Dietitian—has advanced preparation in dietetics and research techniques, plans, investigates, interprets, evaluates, applies and expands knowledge in one or more phases of dietitics and communicates findings through reports and publications.

Teaching Dietitian—has advanced preparation in dietetics or education, plans, conducts, and evaluates educational programs in one or more dietetic subject matter areas.

BIBLIOGRAPHY

Baird, Shirley Chaska, Ed. D., R.D., and Sylvester, Joan, Ph.D.: *Role Delineation and Verification for Entry-Level Positions in Foodservice Systems Management.* Chicago, The American Dietetic Association, 1983.

Baird, Shirley Chaska, Ed. D., R.D., and Sylvester, Joan, Ph.D.: *Role Delineation and Verification for Entry-Level Positions in Community Dietetics.* Chicago, The American Dietetic Association, 1983.

Baird, Shirley Chaska, Ed. D., R.D., Burrelli, Joan, Ph.D., and Flack, Hope, M.A.: *Role Delineation and Verification for Entry-Level Positions in Clinical Dietetics.* Chicago, The American Dietetic Association, 1984.

Position Paper on Recommended Salaries and Employment Practices for Members of the American Dietetic Association, *J. Am. Diet. Assoc.* 78:62, 1981.

Willard, Mervyn D., M.D.: *Nutrition for the Practicing Physician.* Menlo Park, California, Addison–Wesley Publishing Company, 1982.

COORDINATED UNDERGRADUATE PROGRAMS

The Coordinated Undergraduate Program is an accelerated dietetic program that combines didactic and clinical experience within a four-year baccalaureate program.

Each program is accredited by the Commission on Accreditation of ADA and includes an approved Plan IV academic program. The area of emphasis (general, management, clinical, or community) is compatible with the resources available to the program, especially the clinical facilities and faculty experience.

Following is a list of the 66 currently accredited coordinated undergraduate programs.

ALABAMA
Auburn University
Auburn University 36849

The University of Alabama
University 35486

Tuskegee Institute
Tuskegee 36088

CALIFORNIA
Univ. of Calif., Berkeley
Berkeley 94720

Calif. St. Univ., Los
 Angeles
Los Angeles 90032

Loma Linda University
Loma Linda 92350

CONNECTICUT
University of Connecticut
Storrs 06268

Saint Joseph College
W. Hartford 06117

DELAWARE
University of Delaware
Newark 19711

DISTRICT OF COLUMBIA
Howard University
Washington 20059

FLORIDA
University of Florida
Gainesville 32610

Fla. International Univ.
Miami 33199

GEORGIA
Georgia State University
Atlanta 30303

IDAHO
Univ. of Idaho/Eastern
   Washington
Moscow 83843

ILLINOIS
Chicago State University
Chicago 60628

Northern Illinois Univ.
Dekalb 60115–2854

Univ. of Illinois at
   Chicago
Chicago 60612

INDIANA
Indiana State University
Terre Haute 47809

Purdue University
W. Lafayette 47907

IOWA
Iowa State University
Ames 50011

KANSAS
Kansas State University
Manhattan 66506

KENTUCKY
Univ. of Kentucky
Lexington 40506

Spaulding College
Louisville 40203

LOUISIANA
Louisiana University
Ruston 71272

MARYLAND
Hood College
Frederick 21701

MASSACHUSETTS
Framingham State College
Framingham 01701

MICHIGAN
Andrews University
Berrien Springs 49103

Wayne State University
Detroit 48202

Mercy College of Detroit
Detroit 48219

Eastern Michigan Univ.
Ypsilanti 48197

MINNESOTA
University of Minnesota
St. Paul 55108

MISSISSIPPI
Univ. of South. Mississippi
Hattiesburg 39406

MISSOURI
Univ. of Missouri–Columbia
Columbia 65211

NEW YORK
State University College
 at Buffalo
Buffalo 14222

Syracuse University
Syracuse 13210

Rochester Institute of
 Technology
Rochester 14623

NORTH CAROLINA
East Carolina University
Greenville 27834

NORTH DAKOTA
North Dakota St. Univ.
Fargo 58105

Univ. of North Dakota
Grand Forks 58202

OHIO
The Univ. of Akron
Akron 44325

Case Western Reserve Univ.
Cleveland 44106

The Ohio State University
Columbus 43210

OKLAHOMA
Univ. of Oklahoma Health
 Sciences Center
Oklahoma City 73190

PENNSYLVANIA
Pennsylvania Consortium
Maryhurst College
Erie 16546

Villa Maria College
Erie 16505

Drexel University
Philadelphia 19104

Marywood College
Scranton 18509

Edinboro Univ. of
 Pennsylvania
Edinboro 16444

Seton Hill College
Greensburg 15601

University of Pittsburgh
Pittsburgh 15260

SOUTH CAROLINA
Winthrop College
Rock Hill 29733

SOUTH DAKOTA
South Dakota St. Univ.
Brookings 57007–0497

TENNESSEE
The Univ. of Tennessee
Knoxville 37996–1900

TEXAS
The University of Texas
   at Austin
Austin 78712

University of Texas Health
   Science Center at
   Dallas
Dallas 75235

Texas Woman's University
Denton 76204

Univ. of Texas Health
   Science Center at
   Houston
Houston 77225

Texas Christian University
Forth Worth 76129

UTAH
Utah State University
Logan 84322

Brigham Young University
Provo 84602

VIRGINIA
Virginia Polytechnic Inst.
   and State University
Blacksburg 24061

WASHINGTON
Eastern Washington Univ./
   Univ. of Idaho
   Consortium
Cheney 99004

Washington State Univ.
Pullman 99164–2032

WISCONSIN
Viterbo College
LaCrosse 54601

Mount Mary College
Milwaukee 53222

Univ. of Wisconsin–
   Madison
Madison 53706

REFERENCE

The American Dietetic Association. *Directory of Dietetic Programs, 1985,* pp. 4–7. Chicago, Illinois.

DIETETIC INTERNSHIPS

A Dietetic Internship is a post–baccalaureate clinical experience, six to twelve months in length.

Each dietetic internship is accredited by the Commission on Accreditation of ADA and provides an area of emphasis (general, management, clinical, or community) compatible with the resources available to the program.

Internship appointments are awarded on a competitive basis.

Listed below are the 106 currently accredited dietetic internships.

ALABAMA
University of Alabama
Birmingham 35294

ARIZONA
International Heart Found.
Phoenix 85016

University of Arizona
Tucson 85724

ARKANSAS
Univ. of Arkansas for
  Medical Sciences/College
  of Health Related Prof.
Little Rock 72201

CALIFORNIA
Univ. of California
School of Public Health
Berkeley 94520

Univ. of California
Dept. of Food Services
Berkeley 94720

Fairview State Hospital
Costa Mesa 92626

Memorial Hosp. of Glendale
Glendale 91204

Los Angeles County/Univ.
   of S. California
   Medical Center
Los Angeles 90033

Sutter Community Hospitals
Sacramento 95816

Mercy Hospital and Medical
   Center
San Diego 92103

West Los Angeles VA
   Medical Center
Los Angeles 90073

Porterville State Hospital
Porterville 93257

VA Medical Center
San Diego 92161

Univ. of California–San
   Francisco Hospitals
   and Clinics
San Francisco 94143

COLORADO
Penrose Hospitals
Colorado Springs 80933

CONNECTICUT
Yale–New Haven Hospital
New Haven 06504

DISTRICT OF COLUMBIA
Malcolm Grow USAF Medical
   Center
Washington 20331

Walter Reed Army Medical
   Center
Washington 20307

FLORIDA
University of Florida
Gainesville 32611

James A. Haley VA Hosp.
Tampa 33612

Jackson Memorial Hospital
Miami 33136

GEORGIA
Emory University
Atlanta 30303

University Hospital
Augusta 30910

Georgia Baptist Medical
   Center
Atlanta 30312

ILLINOIS
Cook County Hospital
Chicago 60612

Ingalls Mem. Hospital
Harvey 60426

Lutheran Gen. Hospital
Park Ridge 60068

St. John's Hospital
Springfield 62769

Rush–Presbyterian St.
   Luke's Med. Center
Chicago 60612

Edward Hines, Jr. VA Hosp.
Hines 60141

Saint Francis Med. Center
Peoria 61637

INDIANA
Indiana Univ. Med. Center
Indianapolis 46223

Methodist Hospital of
   Indiana, Inc.
Indianapolis 46206

IOWA
The Univ. of Iowa Hospitals
   and Clinics
Iowa City 52242

KANSAS
Univ. of Kansas College of
   Health Sciences and
   Hospital
Kansas City 66103

KENTUCKY
Univ. of Kentucky Medical
   Center
Lexington 40536–0084

LOUISIANA
Alton Ochsner Medical
   Foundation
New Orleans 70121

Touro Infirmary
New Orleans 70115

MARYLAND
Maryland State Dept. of
   Health and Mental
   Hygiene
Baltimore 21201

Mercy Hospital, Inc.
Baltimore 21202

MASSACHUSETTS
Beth Israel Hospital
Boston 02215

Massachusetts Gen. Hosp.
Boston 02114

Brigham and Women's
   Hospital
Boston 02115

Frances Stern Nutrition
   Center
Boston 02111

New England Deaconess
   Hospital
Boston 02215

Mount Auburn Hospital
Cambridge 02238

MICHIGAN
Harper Hospital
Detroit 48201

Henry Ford Hospital
Detroit 48202

Detroit Health Dept.
Detroit 48202

Hurley Medical Center
Flint 48502

Tri–City Dietetic
   Internship
Saginaw 48602

MINNESOTA
Univ. of Minnesota
   Hospitals and Clinics
Minneapolis 55455

Saint Mary's Hospital
Rochester 55902

St. Paul Ramsey Medical
  Center
St. Paul 55101

MISSOURI
Barnes Hospital
St. Louis 63110

VA Medical Center
St. Louis 63125

St. Louis University
St. Louis 63104

NEBRASKA
Univ. of Nebraska-Lincoln
Lincoln 68583-0806

Univ. of Nebraska Medical
  Center
Omaha 68105

NEW JERSEY
VA Medical Center
East Orange 07019

Raritan Bay Med. Center
Perth Amboy 08861

Univ. of Medicine and
  Dentistry of NJ School
  of Health Related
  Professions
Newark 07103

NEW YORK
VA Medical Center
Bronx 10468

The New York Hospital
New York 10021

United Health Services,
  Inc.
Johnson City 13790

Westchester County Medical
  Center
Vahalla 10595

OHIO
The Christ Hospital
Cincinnati 45219

Good Samaritan Hospital
Cincinnati 45220

Univ. Hospitals of
  Cleveland
Cleveland 44106

Cleveland Metropolitan
  General/Highland
  View Hospital
Cleveland 44109

Miami Valley Hospital
Dayton 45409

Univ. of Cincinnati Hosp.
Cincinnati 45267-0716

Case Western Reserve Univ.
Cleveland 44106

Cleveland VA Medical
  Center
Cleveland 44106

Saint Luke's Hospital
Cleveland 44102

Riverside Methodist Hosp.
Columbus 43214

OKLAHOMA
Oklahoma State University
Stillwater 74078

Saint Francis Hospital
Tulsa 74136

OREGON
Oregon Health Sciences Univ.
Portland 97201

PENNSYLVANIA
Wood Enterprises/Lehigh
Valley Hosp. Center
Allentown 18103

Shadyside Hospital
Pittsburgh 15232

Johnstown Area Dietetic
Internship
Johnstown 15901

York Hospital
York 17405

PUERTO RICO
Medical Sciences Campus
Univ. of Puerto Rico
San Juan 00936

Health Department
San Juan 00936

Univ. of Puerto Rico and
VA Hospital
San Juan 00931

RHODE ISLAND
Rhode Island Hospital
Providence 02902

SOUTH DAKOTA
McKennan Hospital
Sioux Falls 57101

TENNESSEE
National Health Corp.
Murfreesboro 37130

Vanderbilt University
Medical Center
Nashville 37232

Univ. of Tennessee Center
for Health Sciences
Memphis 38105

TEXAS
Texas A & M Univ.
College Station 77843

Presbyterian Hospital of
Dallas
Dallas 75225

VA Medical Center
Houston 77211

Baylor Univ. Med. Center
Dallas 75246

Brooke Army Medical Center
Fort Sam Houston 78234

Texas Woman's University
Houston 77030

Baptist Memorial Hospital
System
San Antonio 78286

UTAH
VA Medical Center (1200)
Salt Lake City 84148

VIRGINIA
Univ. of Virginia Hospital
Charlottesville 22908

Medical College of
   Virginia Hospitals
Richmond 23298–0001

WEST VIRGINIA
West Virginia Univ. Hosp.
Morgantown 26506

WISCONSIN
Univ. of Wisconsin Hospital
   and Clinics
Madison 53792

Milwaukee Public Schools
Milwaukee 53210

St. Luke's Hospital
Milwaukee 53215

REFERENCES

The American Dietetic Association. *Directory of Dietetic Programs, 1985,* pp. 8–13. Chicago, Illinois.

DIETETIC TECHNICIAL PROGRAMS

The Dietetic Technician Program is a two–year program leading to an associate degree. The program is a combination of didactic and clinical experiences.

Following is a list of the 80 dietetic technician programs approved by The American Dietetic Association.

ALABAMA
University of Alabama
Birmingham 35294

ARIZONA
Central Arizona College
Coolidge 85228

CALIFORNIA
Chaffey Community College
Alta Lorna 91762

Bakersfield College
Bakersfield 93305

Long Beach City College
Long Beach 90808

Mission College
Santa Clara 95054

Pacific Union College
Angwin 94508

Orange Coast College
Costa Mesa 92626–0120

Los Angeles City College
Los Angeles 90029

COLORADO
Pikes Peak Comm. College
Colorado Springs 80906

Front Range Comm. College
Westminster 80030

CONNECTICUT
South Central Comm. College
New Haven 06511

University of New Haven
West Haven 06516

127

Briarwood College
Southington 06489

FLORIDA
Broward Community College
Fort Lauderdale 33314

Palm Beach Jr. College
Lake Worth 33461

Valencia Community College
Orlando 32802

Florida Junior College
Jacksonville 32210

Miami Dade Comm. College
Miami 33132

Pensacola Junior College
Pensacola 32504

ILLINOIS
Malcolm X College
Chicago 60612

Wm. Rainey Harper College
Palatine 60067

INDIANA
University of Evansville
Evansville 47702

Ball State University
Muncie 47306

Marion College
Indianapolis 46222

Purdue University
West Lafayette 47907

KANSAS
Coffeyville Comm. College
Coffeyville 67337

Butler County Community
   College and Wichita
   Area Vo–Tech School
Wichita 67202

KENTUCKY
Murray State University
Murray 42071

Eastern Kentucky Univ.
Richmond 40475–0936

LOUISIANA
Louisiana Tech University
Ruston 71272

MAINE
Univ. of Maine at
   Farmington
Farmington 04938

Southern Maine Vo–Tech
   Institute
South Portland 04106

MARYLAND
Comm. College of Baltimore
Baltimore 21215

Montgomery College
Rockville 20850

MASSACHUSETTS

Laboure Junior College
Boston 02124

Holyoke Comm. College
Holyoke 01040

MICHIGAN
Mercy College of Detroit
Detroit 48219

Oakland Comm. College
Farmington Hills 48018

Wayne County Comm. College
Detroit 48228

MINNESOTA
Normandale Comm. College
Bloomingdale 55431

Lakewood Comm. College
White Bear Lake 55110

Univ. of Minnesota
Crookston 56716

MISSOURI
St. Louis Comm. College at
Florissant Valley
St. Louis 63135

NEBRASKA
Central Comm. College
Hastings 68901

Southeast Comm. College
Lincoln 68520

NEW JERSEY
Camden Comm. College
Blackwood 08012

Middlesex County College
Edison 08818

NEW YORK
Erie Comm. College
Buffalo 14221

LaGuardia Comm. College
Long Island City 11101

New York University
New York 10003

State Univ. of New York
Cobleskill 12043

New York State Agric. and
Technical College
Morrisville 13408

Dutchess Comm. College
Poughkeepsie 12601

Suffolk County Comm.
College
Riverhead 11901

Westchester Comm. College
Vahalla 10595

Rockland Comm. College
Suffern 10901

OHIO
Cincinnati Tech. College
Cincinnati 45223

Columbus Tech. Institute
Columbus 43216

Hocking Tech. College
Nelsonville 45764

Cuyahoga Comm. College
Cleveland 44115

Kettering College of
Medical Arts
Kettering 45429

Youngstown State Univ.
Youngstown 44555

OREGON
Portland Comm. College
Portland 97219

PENNSYLVANIA
Harrisburg Area Community
   College
Harrisburg 17110

Comm. College of Allegheny
   County
Pittsburgh 15212

Williamsport Area Comm.
   College
Williamsport 17701

Community College of
   Philadelphia
Philadelphia 19130

The Pennsylvania State
   University
University Park 16802

TENNESSEE
Shelby State Comm. College
Memphis 38174–0568

TEXAS
El Paso Comm. College
El Paso 79998

Tarrant County Jr. College
Fort Worth 76119

Southwestern Adventist
   College
Keene 76059

VIRGINIA
Northern Virginia Comm.
Annadale 22003

Tidewater Comm. College
Virginia Beach 23456

WASHINGTON
Shoreline Comm. College
Seattle 98133

WISCONSIN
Madison Area Tech. College
Madison 53703

Milwaukee Area Tech.
   College
Milwaukee 53203

Cardinal Stritch College
Milwaukee 53217

Mid–State Tech. Institute
Wisconsin Rapids 54494

REFERENCES

The American Dietetic Association. *Directory of Dietetic Programs, 1985,* pp. 14–17. Chicago, Illinois.

PLAN IV PROGRAMS

Plan IV Program is a term used by The American Dietetic Association to describe the competency–based program approved as meeting the academic component of the eligibility requirements to take the registration examination for dietitians as well as the academic requirement for membership in The American Dietetic Association.

Following is a list of the 272 Plan IV programs approved by The American Dietetic Association. It should be noted that additional programs are approved on a continuing basis, and you should check with the ADA when you are ready to make your plans.

ALABAMA
Auburn University
Auburn 36849

Oakwood College
Huntsville 35896

Sanford University
Birmingham 35229

Jacksonville St. Univ.
Jacksonville 36265

Univ. of Montevallo
Montevallo 35115

The Univ. of Alabama
University 35486

Alabama A & M Univ.
Normal 35762

ARIZONA
Northern Arizona Univ.
Flagstaff 86001

University of Arizona
Tucson
85721

Arizona State University
Tempe 85261

ARKANSAS
Quachita Baptist Univ.
Arkadelphia 71923

Univ. of Central Arkansas
Conway 72032

University of Arkansas
Fayetteville 72701

Univ. of Arkansas
Pine Bluff 71601

Harding University
Searcy 72143

CALIFORNIA
Pacific Union College
Angwin 94508

Univ. of Calif., Berkeley
Berkeley 94720

Univ. of Calif., Davis
Davis 95616

California St. Univ.
Long Beach 90840

Pepperdine University
Malibu 90265

Calif. St. Poly. Univ.
Pomona 91768

College of Notre Dame
Belmont 94002

California St. Univ.
Chico 95929

California St. Univ.
Fresno 93740

California St. Univ.
Los Angeles 90032

California St. Univ.
Northridge 91330

San Diego State Univ.
San Diego 92182–0282

San Francisco St. Univ.
San Francisco 94132

Calif. Poly. St. Univ.
San Luis Obispo 93401

San Jose State Univ.
San Jose 95112

Whittier College
Whittier 90608

COLORADO
Colorado State Univ.
Fort Collins 80523

Univ. of Northern Colorado
Greeley 80639

CONNECTICUT
Albertus Magnus College
New Haven 06511

St. Joseph's College
West Hartford 06117

Univ. of Connecticut
Storrs 06268

Univ. of New Haven
West Haven 06516

DELAWARE
Univ. of Delaware
Newark 19716

DISTRICT OF COLUMBIA
Howard Univ.
Washington 20059

Univ. of the District of
  Columbia
Washington 20001

FLORIDA
Univ. of Florida
Gainesville 32611

The Univ. of W. Florida
Pensacola 32504

Florida Int'l Univ.
Miami 33199

Florida State Univ.
Tallahassee 32306

GEORGIA
Univ. of Georgia
Athens 30602

Emory Univ. School of
  Medicine
Atlanta 30303

Clark College
Atlanta 30314

Fort Valley State College
Fort Valley 31030

Savannah State College
Savannah 31404

Georgia College
Milledgeville 31061

Georgia Southern College
Statesboro 30460-8034

HAWAII
Univ. of Hawaii-Manoa
Honolulu 96822

IDAHO
Idaho State Univ.
Pocatello 83209

ILLINOIS
Southern Illinois Univ.
Carbondale 62901

Chicago State Univ.
Chicago 60628

Eastern Illinois Univ.
Charleston 61920

Mundelein College
Chicago 60660

Northern Illinois Univ.
Dekalb 60115-2854

Illinois Benedictine Col.
Lisle 60532

Illinois State Univ.
Normal 61761

Rosary College
River Forest 60305

Olivet Nazarene College
Kankakee 60901

Western Illinois Univ.
Macomb 61455

Bradley Univ.
Peoria 61625

Univ. of Illinois
Urbana 61801

INDIANA
Marian College
Indianapolis 46222

St. Mary of the Woods Col.
St. Mary of the Woods 47876

Valparaiso Univ.
Valparaiso 46383

Ball State Univ.
Muncie 47306

Indiana State Univ.
Terre Haute 47809

Purdue Univ.
Dept. of Foods and Nutr.
West Lafayette 47907

Purdue Univ.
Dept. of Rest., Hotel and
   Institutional Mgmt.
West Lafayette 47907

IOWA
Iowa State Univ.
Dept. of Food and Nutr.
Ames 50011

Univ. of Northern Iowa
Cedar Ralls 50614

Univ. of Iowa
Iowa City 52242

Iowa State Univ.
Dept. of Hotel, Rest. and
   Institution Mgmt.
Ames 50011

Marycrest College
Davenport 52804

Iowa Wesleyan College
Mount Pleasant 52641

KANSAS
Benedictine College
Atchison 66002

Fort Hays State Univ.
Hays 67601

Saint Mary College
Leavenworth 66048

Kansas State Univ.
Dept. of Diet., Rest. and
   Institutional Mgmt.
Justine Hall 104
Manhattan 66506

Kansas State Univ.
Dept. of Diet., Rest. and
   Institutional Mgmt.
Justin Hall 106
Manhattan 66506

Kansas State Univ.
College of Home Economics
Manhattan 66506

KENTUCKY
Berea College
Berea 40404

Kentucky State Univ.
Frankfort 40601

Univ. of Louisville
Louisville 40292

Murray State Univ.
Murray 42071

Western Kentucky Univ.
Bowling Green 42101

Univ. of Kentucky
Lexington 40506

Morehead State Univ.
Morehead 40351

Eastern Kentucky Univ.
Richmond 40475

LOUISIANA
Louisiana State Univ.
Baton Rouge 70803

Grambling College
Grambling 71245

Univ. of S. W. Louisiana
Lafayette 70504

Northwestern State Univ.
Natchitoches 71497

Nicholls State Univ.
Thibodaux 70310

Southern Univ.
Baton Rouge 70813

S. Eastern Louisiana Univ.
Hammond 70402

Northeast Louisiana Univ.
Monroe 71209

Louisiana Tech Univ.
Ruston 71272

MAINE
Univ. of Maine
Orono 04469

MARYLAND
Morgan State Univ.
Baltimore 21239

Hood College
Frederick 21701

Univ. of Maryland
College Park 20742

Univ. of Maryland,
   Eastern Shore
Princess Anne 21853

MASSACHUSETTS
Univ. of Massachusetts
Amherst 01003

Framingham State College
Framingham 01701

Simmons College
Boston 02115

Atlantic Union College
South Lancaster 01561

MICHIGAN
Marygrove College
Detroit 48221

Wayne State Univ.
Detroit 48202

Michigan State Univ.
East Lansing 48824–1030

Madonna College
Livonia 48150

Central Michigan Univ.
Mt. Pleasant 48859

Western Michigan Univ.
Kalamazoo 49008

Northern Michigan Univ.
Marquette 49855

MINNESOTA
College of St. Scholastica
Duluth 55811

Concordia College
Moorhead 56560

The Col. of St. Catherine
St. Paul 55105

College of Saint Teresa
Winona 55987

Mankato State Univ.
Mankato 56001

College of St. Benedict
St. Joseph 56374

Univ. of Minnesota
St. Paul 55108

MISSISSIPPI
Mississippi College
Clinton 39058

Univ. of S. Mississippi
Hattiesburg 39406

Mississippi State Univ.
Mississippi State 39762

Mississippi Univ. for
Women
Columbus 39701

Alcorn State Univ.
Lorman 39096

Univ. of Mississippi
University 38677

MISSOURI
Southwest Baptist Univ.
Bolivar 65613

Univ. of Missouri–Columbia
Columbia 65211

N. W. Missouri State Univ.
Maryville 64468

S. E. Missouri State Univ.
Cape Girardeau 63701

Lincoln Univ.
Jefferson City 65101

The School of the Ozarks
Point Lookout 65726

Drury College
Springfield 65802

Fontbonne College
St. Louis 63105

S. W. Missouri State Univ.
Springfield 65804

Central Missouri State
    Univ.
Warrensburg 64093

MONTANA
Montana State Univ.
Bozeman 59717

Univ. of Montana
Missoula 59812

Nebraska
Kearney State College
Kearney 68849–0512

Univ. of Nebraska–Omaha
Omaha 68182–0211

Univ. of Nebraska–Lincoln
Lincoln 68583–0806

NEVADA
Univ. of Nevada
Reno 89557

NEW HAMPSHIRE
Univ. of New Hampshire
Durham 03824

Rivier College
Nashua 03060

Keene State College
Keene 03431

NEW JERSEY
College of St. Elizabeth
Convent Station 07961

Rutgers Univ.
New Brunswick 08903

Glassboro State College
Glassboro 08028

Montclair State College
Upper Montclair 07043

NEW MEXICO
Univ. of New Mexico
Albuquerque 87131

New Mexico State Univ.
Las Cruces 88003

NEW YORK
Herbert H. Lehman College
Bronx 10468

Pratt Institute
Brooklyn 11205

Queens College
Flushing 11367

Hunter College
New York 10010

State Univ. of New York
Oneonta 13820

Rochester Inst. of Tech.
Rochester 14623

Marymont College
Tarrytown 10591

Brooklyn College
Brooklyn 11210

St. Univ. Col. at Buffalo
Buffalo 14222

Cornell University
Ithaca 14853

New York University
New York 10003

Plattsburg State Univ.
Plattsburg 12901

Syracuse University
Syracuse 13210

Russell Sage College
Troy 12180

NORTH CAROLINA
Appalachian State Univ.
Boone 28608

Western Carolina Univ.
Cullowhee 28723

Bennett College
Greensboro 27401-3239

Univ. of North Carolina
Greensboro 27412-5001

Meredith College
Raleigh 27607-5298

Univ. of North Carolina
Chapel Hill 27514

North Carolina Cent. Univ.
Durham 27707

N. Carolina A&T St. Univ.
Greensboro 27411

East Carolina University
Greenville 27834

Salem College
Winston Salem 27108

NORTH DAKOTA
North Dakota St. Univ.
Fargo 58105

OHIO
The Univ. of Akron
Akron 44325

Bowling Green St. Univ.
Bowling Green 43403

Univ. of Cincinnati
Cincinnati 45221

The Ohio State Univ.
Columbus 43210

Kent State University
Kent 44242

Miami University
Oxford 45056

Youngstown State Univ.
Youngstown 44555

Ohio University
Athens 45701

Case Western Reserve Univ.
Cleveland 44106

Notre Dame College
Cleveland 44121

University of Dayton
Dayton 45469

Col. of Mount St. Joseph
Mount St. Joseph 45051

Otterbein College
Westerville 43085

OKLAHOMA
Central State University
Edmond 73034

Oklahoma State University
Stillwater 74078

Univ. of Oklahoma
Norman 73019

OREGON
Oregon State University
Corvallis 97331

PENNSYLVANIA
Cheyney St. Univ. of Penna.
Cheyney 19319

Messiah College
Grantham 17027

Immaculata College
Immaculata 19345

College Misericordia
Dallas 18612

Seton Hill College
Greensburg 15601

Indiana Univ. of Penna.
Indiana 15705

Mansfield Univ. of PA
Mansfield 16933

University of Pittsburgh
Pittsburgh 15260

Marywood College
Scranton 18509

The Penna. St. Univ.
Nutrition Program
University Park 16802

Drexel University
Philadelphia 19104

Albright College
Reading 19603

Shippensburg University
Shippensburg 17257

PUERTO RICO
Univ. of Puerto Rico and
V. A. Hospital
San Juan 00931

RHODE ISLAND
Univ. of Rhode Island
Kingston 02881–0809

SOUTH CAROLINA
Clemson University
Clemson 29631

Winthrop College
Rock Hill 29733

South Carolina St. College
Orangeburg 29117

SOUTH DAKOTA
South Dakota St. Univ.
Brookings 57007–0497

Mount Marty College
Yankton 57078

TENNESSEE
Tennessee Tech. University
Cookeville 38501

Carson–Newman College
Jefferson City 37760

Univ. of Tennessee
Knoxville 37996–1900

University of Tennessee
Chattanooga 37402

East Tennessee St. Univ.
Johnson City 37614

Univ. of Tennessee
Martin 38238–5045

Memphis St. Univ.
Memphis 38152

David Lipscomb College
Nashville 37203,

Middle Tenn. St. Univ.
Murfreesboro 37132

Tennessee St. Univ.
Nashville 37203

TEXAS
Abilene Christian Univ.
Abilene 79699

Lamar University
Beaumont 77710

Texas A & M Univ.
College Station 77043

North Texas St. Univ.
Denton 76203

Texas Christian Univ.
Fort Worth 76129

The Univ. of Texas
Austin 78712

Un. of Mary Hardin–Baylor
Belton 76513

East Texas St. Univ.
Commerce 75428

Texas Woman's Univ.
Denton 76204

Texas Southern Univ.
Houston 77004

Univ. of Houston
Univ. Park Campus
Houston 77004

Sam Houston St. Univ.
Huntsville 77341

Texas Tech Univ.
Lubbock 79409

Prairie View A & M Univ.
Prairie 77445

Southwest Texas St. Univ.
San Marcos 78666

Univ. of Texas Health
   Science Center
Houston 77225

Texas A & I Univ.
Kingsville 78363

S. F. Austin St. Univ.
Nacogdoches 75962

Incarnate Word College
San Antonio 78209

Baylor University
Waco 76798

UTAH
Utah State University
Logan 84322

Brigham Young University
Provo 84602

The Univ. of Utah
Salt Lake City 84112

VERMONT
University of Vermont
Burlington 05405

VIRGINIA
Virginia Polytech. Inst.
Blacksburg 24061–8398

Eastern Mennonite Col.
Harrisonburg 22801

Virginia State Univ.
Petersburg 23803

Hampton Institute
Hampton 23668

James Madison Univ.
Harrisonburg 22807

Radford University
Radford 24142

WASHINGTON
Central Washington Univ.
Ellensburg 98926

Washington State Univ.
Pullman 99164–2032

Univ. of Washington
Seattle 98195

WEST VIRGINIA
W. Virginia Wesleyan Col.
Buckhannon 26201

West Virginia University
Morgantown 26506–6122

Marshall University
Huntington 25701

WISCONSIN
Univ. of Wisconsin
Human Biology Dept.
Green Bay 54301–7001

Univ. of Wisconsin
Dept. of Food Service
Madison 53706

Univ. of Wisconsin
Stevens Point 54481

Univ. of Wisconsin Dept of Nutr.
  Services
Madison 53706

Univ. of Wisconsin–Stout
Menomonie 54751

Cardinal Stritch College
Milwaukee 53217

WYOMING
University of Wyoming
Laramie 82071

REFERENCE

The American Dietetic Association. *Directory of Dietetic Programs, 1985,* pp. 18–31. Chicago, Illinois.

VGM CAREER BOOKS

OPPORTUNITIES IN

*Available in both
paperback and hardbound
editions*

Accounting Careers
Acting Careers
Advertising Careers
Airline Careers
Animal and Pet Care
Appraising Valuation Science
Architecture
Automotive Service
Banking
Beauty Culture
Biological Sciences
Book Publishing
Broadcasting Careers
Building Construction
 Trades
Business Management
Cable Television
Carpentry
Chemical Engineering
Chemistry
Chiropractic Health Care
Civil Engineering
Commercial Art and Graphic
 Design
Computer Science Careers
Counseling & Development
Dance
Data Processing Careers
Dental Care
Drafting Careers
Electrical Trades
Electronic and Electrical
 Engineering
Energy Careers
Engineering Technology
Environmental Careers
Fashion
Federal Government Careers
Film Careers
Financial Careers
Fire Protection Services
Food Services
Foreign Language Careers

Forestry Careers
Free Lance Writing
Government Service
Graphic Communications
Health and
 Medical Careers
Hospital Administration
Hotel & Motel Management
Industrial Design
Interior Design
Journalism Careers
Landscape Architecture
Law Careers
Law Enforcement and
 Criminal Justice
Library and Information
 Science
Machine Shop Trades
Magazine Publishing
Management
Marine & Maritime
Materials Science
Mechanical Engineering
Microelectronics
Modeling Careers
Music Careers
Nursing Careers
Nutrition Careers
Occupational Therapy
Office Occupations
Opticianry
Optometry
Packaging Science
Paralegal Careers
Paramedical Careers
Personnel Management
Pharmacy Careers
Photography
Physical Therapy
Podiatric Medicine
Printing Careers
Psychiatry
Psychology
Public Relations Careers
Real Estate
Recreation and Leisure
Refrigeration and
 Air Conditioning

Religious Service
Sales & Marketing
Secretarial Careers
Securities Industry
Sports & Athletics
Sports Medicine
State and Local Government
Teaching Careers
Technical
 Communications
Telecommunications
Theatrical Design
 & Production
Transportation
Travel Careers
Veterinary Medicine
Word Processing
Writing Careers
Your Own Service Business

WOMEN IN

*Available in both
paperback and hardbound
editions*

Communications
Engineering
Finance
Government
Management
Science
Their Own Business

CAREER PLANNING

How to Land a Better Job
How to Write a Winning
 Résumé
Life Plan
Planning Your College
 Education
Planning Your Military Career
Planning Your Own Home
 Business

SURVIVAL GUIDES

High School Survival Guide
College Survival Guide

 VGM Career Horizons

A Division of National Textbook Company
4255 West Touhy Avenue
Lincolnwood, Illinois 60646-1975 U.S.A.